LUNG CANCER THERAPY ANNUAL 3

Heine H Hansen, MD, FRCP
Professor of Medical Oncology
The Finsen Center, National University Hospital, Copenhagen, Denmark

Paul A Bunn Jr, MD
Grohne/Stapp Professor and Director
University of Colorado Cancer Center, Denver, CO, USA

Karen Kelly, MD
Associate Professor of Medicine
University of Colorado Cancer Center, Denver, CO, USA

With contributions from
David Raben, MD, PhD
Associate Professor of Radiation Oncology, University of Colorado Cancer Center
Robert M. Jotte, MD, PhD
Director of Thoracic Oncology, Denver Division Rocky Mountain Cancer Centers

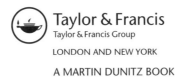

Taylor & Francis
Taylor & Francis Group

LONDON AND NEW YORK

A MARTIN DUNITZ BOOK

© 2003, 2004 Taylor & Francis, an imprint of the Taylor & Francis Group

First published in the United Kingdom in 2003
by Taylor & Francis, an imprint of the Taylor and Francis Group, 11 New Fetter Lane,
London EC4P 4EE

Tel.:   +44 (0) 20 7583 9855
Fax.:   +44 (0) 20 7842 2298
E-mail: info@dunitz.co.uk
Website: http://www.dunitz.co.uk

Reprinted twice in 2004

A CIP record for this book is available from the British Library.

Library of Congress Cataloging-in-Publication Data

Data available on application

ISBN 1 84184 302 4

Distributed in North and South America by

Taylor & Francis
2000 NW Corporate Blvd
Boca Raton, FL 33431, USA

Within Continental USA
Tel.: 800 272 7737; Fax.: 800 374 3401
Outside Continental USA
Tel.: 561 994 0555; Fax.: 561 361 6018
E-mail: orders@crcpress.com

Distributed in the rest of the world by
Thomson Publishing Services
Cheriton House
North Way
Andover, Hampshire SP10 5BE, UK
Tel.: +44 (0)1264 332424
E-mail: salesorder.tandf@thomsonpublishingservices.co.uk

Composition by EXPO Holdings, Malaysia
Printed and bound by Biddles, Kings Lynn, UK

Contents

Preface

The purpose of this third edition of Lung Cancer Therapy Annual remains the same as for the previous issues: to brief the oncology community about the most recent developments in lung cancer by reviewing the literature from the last year, with emphasis on the therapeutic aspects, and to offer an update of the impact that this information will have on the day-to-day management of lung cancer patients.

The editors are grateful to their co-authors whose scholarship has contributed to the quality of the book. Special thanks are due to Dr. David Raben and Dr. Robert M. Jotte, who co-authored the chapter on non-small cell lung cancer. The editors gratefully acknowledge the cooperation and help of Alison Campbell and Robert Peden of Martin Dunitz Ltd. The interest and help of the publisher is greatly appreciated.

Heine H. Hansen, M.D.
Paul A. Bunn, Jr., M.D.
Karen Kelly, M.D.

1
Introduction

Worldwide, smoking kills more than 4 million people each year, and this figure is increasing.[1] It is therefore not surprising that the number of patients with lung cancer – a disease that has been clearly and unambiguously linked to tobacco consumption, especially cigarette smoking – is also on the rise. Lung cancer accounts for 12.8% of cancer cases and 17.8% of cancer deaths in the world.

In spite of recent strides in the understanding of the molecular biology of lung cancer,[2] new tools for early detection and screening, and the development of novel cancer and precancer therapies, tobacco control remains the main target for reducing the incidence of lung cancer. The establishment of global anti-tobacco policy has been strengthened in recent years, with the most effective elements being increases in the tax on cigarettes, but this varies considerably; for instance, in the EU, a total ban on cigarette advertisement, no-smoking policies at work and in public places, and prominent warnings on cigarette packages are employed.[3] Unifying global tobacco control efforts have recently been spearheaded by the WHO's Tobacco-Free Initiative, with the establishment of World No Tobacco Day on May 31, partnered with such organizations as UNICEF, the World Bank, the US Centers for Disease Control and Prevention, and the US Environmental Protection Agency.[4] Also, physicians, including oncologists, are getting increasingly involved in these tasks, and evidenced-based recommendations on the treatment of tobacco dependence were published by the WHO in June 2001.[5–7]

However, the opponent in this battle is very strong. The tobacco industry's yearly income is more than US$400 billion, and is only exceeded by the gross national product in 15 countries.[8,9]

A major problem in tobacco control efforts has been the development of an appropriate set of international standards to regulate tobacco products and to inform the public correctly about the nicotine intake per cigarette smoked.[10,11] Recent investigations have revealed that yields of tar and nicotine for machine-smoked cigarettes provide a very poor guide to smokers' exposure and that official tar tests are misleading.[12,13] Furthermore, tobacco campaigns in 2001 have undermined healthcare initiatives ranging from smoke-free areas to cigarette advertisement bans, for example in Switzerland.[14] Although the tar and nicotine during the last 40 years have decreased along with the levels of

1

polycyclic aromatic hydrocarbons, the levels of specific nitrosamines have increased. Evidence is emerging that these products cause various types of DNA damage, including damage to tumor suppressor gene and oncogenes.[15] Furthermore, reports have been published that metabolites of the tobacco-specific lung carcinogen 4-methylnitrosoamino)-1-(3-pyridyl)-1-butanone in non-smoking women exposed to environmental tobacco smoke make an important contribution that explains the excess risk for lung cancer in this cohort of patients.[16]

New scientific information is thus appearing linking tobacco consumption to lung cancer, and tobacco control efforts are slowly gaining momentum world-wide, with new smoking laws in such countries as India and Kenya,[17–19] offering renewed optimism. However, irrespective of these efforts, lung cancer will remain a major burden on the healthcare system globally for many decades to come.

REFERENCES

1. Twombly R. World Health Organization takes on "Tobacco Epedèmic". J NATC Cancer Inst 2002; **94**: 644–6.

2. Sozzi G. Molecular biology of lung cancer. Eur J Cancer 2001; **37** (Suppl 7): S63–S72.

3. Montes A, Villalbi JR. The price of cigarettes in the European Union. Tobacco Control 2001; **10**: 135–6.

4. McCann J. Anti-smoking efforts seeks global implementation. J Natl Cancer Inst 2000; **92**: 523–4.

5. Doctors and Tobacco. Tobacco Control Resource Centre, European Commission 2000.

6. World Health Organization. Evidence Based Recommendations on the Treatment of Tobacco Dependence. European Partnership to Reduce Tobacco Dependence. Geneva: World Health Organization, 2001.

7. Carter CL, Key J, March L, Graves K. Contemporary perspectives in tobacco cessation: what oncologists need to know. Oncologist 2001; **6**: 496–505.

8. Tønnesen P, Vermeire PA. Promoting a future without tobaco:

also a continuing task for respiratory medicine in Europe. Eur Respir J 2000; **16**: 1031–4.

9. Argyropoulos P. Advertisement and education of the public. Abstract Book, 4th International Congress on Lung Cancer, Halkidiki, Greece. Hellenic Society Against Lung Cancer, 2001.

10. Jarvis MJ, Boreham R, Primatesta P et al. Nicotine yield from machine-smoked cigarettes and nicotine intakes in smokers: evidence from a representataive population survey. J Natl Cancer Inst 2001; **93**: 134–8.

11. Han A. Challenging public health acceptability of current international standards on tobacco products: paving the way for strengthened cooperation. Tobacco Control 2001; **10**: 105–7.

12. Peeler CL, Butters GR. Re: It's time for a change: cigarette smokers deserve meaningful information about their cigarettes. Correspondence. J Natl Cancer Inst 2000; **92**: 842–3.

13. Kozloski LT, O'Connor RJ. Official cigarette tar tests are misleading: use a two-stage, compensating test. Lancet 2000; **355**: 2159–61.

14. Kapp C. Tobacco campaigns 'undermined' in Switzerland. *Lancet* 2001; 357: 208.

15. Shields PG. Epidemiology of tobacco carcinogenesis. *Curr Oncol Rep* 2000; 2: 257–62.

16. Chobanyan NS, Nersesyan AK. Re: Metabolites of a tobacco-specific lung carcinogen in nonsmoking women exposed to environmental tobacco smoke. Correspondence. *J Natl Cancer Inst* 2001; 93: 1575–6.

17. Lancet Oncology. India's new smoking laws – progress or politics? *Lancet Oncol* 2001; 2: 123.

18. Vaidya JS. India's new smoking laws. *Lancet Oncol* 2001; 2: 198.

19. Kapp C. Health, trade, and industry officials set to debate access to essential drugs. *Lancet* 2001; 357: 1105.

2
Epidemiology

Lung cancer remains the number one cause of cancer deaths in North America and many western European countries, and the disease is rapidly on the rise in the rest of the world, especially southern and eastern Europe[1] and China, but also in other heavily populated countries such as Brazil.[2] Within recent years, the epidemiologic features of lung cancer have changed drastically, being influenced by the fact that relatively more females are smoking today than two to three decades ago. In Brazil, the mortality rate from lung cancer for females rose from 4.8 per 100 000 in 1980 to 11.2 in 1998 (Figure 2.1).

Among youngsters the US Centers for Disease Control and Prevention has analyzed the results of an analysis examining changes in cigarette smoking among high school students in the USA from 1991 to 1999.[3] The results indicate that current smoking among high school students in the USA increased significantly from 27.5% in 1991 to 34.8% in 1999. However, the analysis also suggested that later in the decade, current smoking may have leveled or possibly begun to decline – a rather positive trend. How to reduce smoking among teenagers has been addressed in an editorial by Tønnesen.[4]

The impact of changes in 'tar' yields has been evaluated from population studies, both in the USA and in Australia. In the American study, the US mortality database (1960–1994) for all deaths among Whites in which lung cancer was listed as the underlying cause of death was searched, and surveys from

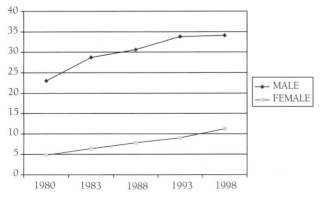

Figure 2.1

Lung cancer crude rates (per 100 000) for mortality, Rio Grande do Sul

1970, 1978–1980, and 1992 were used to estimate the annual number of current and recent smokers in 11 five-year birth cohorts, starting in 1901.[5] The population-based rates of lung cancer mortality were much higher among men than among women across all ages and birth cohorts, reflecting higher smoking rates among men. These differences decreased after being controlled for current and recent smoking within the cohorts, and were slightly increased in women thereafter. The authors conclude that differences in lung cancer death rates across birth cohorts of US men and women primarily reflect differences in the prevalence and duration of smoking in these cohorts. Changes in cigarette design that have greatly reduced tar yields have a relative small effect compared with smoking status and duration of smoking.

An Australian population study showed that lung cancer mortality rates of 20 to 44-year-old Australian women peaked in 1986.[6,7] Age-adjusted mortality rates are lower for women born in the 1950s and 1960s than for women born in the 1940s, despite higher proportions of smokers, younger age of commencement, and longer duration of smoking by age 30 years in the more recent cohorts. Increased smoking has thus not resulted in higher lung cancer mortality for Australian women born in the 1950s and 1960s. Reductions in tar yields of Australian-made cigarettes, which would have affected primarily those born after the 1940s, may be responsible. It will be of interest to see whether future studies shed light on the relation between reduced tar yields and lung cancer mortality.

Other population studies have focused on the association between lung cancer risk and gender, with several studies in the past showing appreciably higher lung cancer risk estimates associated with smoking exposure among men than among women, while other studies in the USA report just the opposite. To elucidate this problem, Kreuzer et al[8] performed a multicenter case–control study in Germany and Italy, but were unable to demonstrate any differences, concluding that for comparable exposure to tobacco smoke, the risk of lung cancer is comparable in women and men.

Siegfried[9] emphasizes that there is still much controversy about whether or not there is an increased lung cancer risk in women across all populations. In Siegfried's review, she suggests that women may be more prone to exposure to a specific lung carcinogen than men and are more susceptible to the adverse effects of tobacco smoke, resulting in more carcinogenic products in women than in men. Finally, she speculates that estrogens may contribute to the development of lung cancer in females.

Other risk factors have been implemented in studies by Darby et al.[10] In a case–control study of 1000 cases and 1500 controls in south-west England, they demonstrated that preformed retinol was associated with an increased risk for lung cancer, while fish liver oil, vitamin pills, carrots, and tomato sauce resulted in a decreased risk.

Kreuzer et al[11] studied lung cancer in lifetime non-smoking men in Germany, and concluded that occupational carcinogens and indoor radon may play a role in some lung cancers in non-smoking men. This was based on interviews of 58 male cases with confirmed primary lung cancer and 803 male controls combined with 1-year radon measurements in the living rooms and bedrooms of the subjects' dwellings.

Finally, Janssen-Heijnen et al[12,13] focused on the trends in incidence of various histologic subtypes based on literature studies comparing data from North America, Australia, New Zealand, and Europe, or from data collected at the Eindhoven Cancer Registry. They concluded that although lung cancer has been decreasing since the 1970s/1980s among men in North America, Australia, New Zealand, and north-western Europe, the age-adjusted rate continues to increase among women in these countries and among both men and women in southern and eastern Europe. These trends follow changes in smoking behavior. The proportion of adenocarcinoma has been increasing over time; the most likely explanation is the shift to low-tar filter cigarettes during the 1960s and 1970s. The use of filters by long-standing smokers generally results in different inhalation behavior, for example taking larger puffs and retaining smoke longer to compensate for the lower nicotine yield of filter cigarettes. The subsequent increased deposits of smoking particles in the bronchioles could enhance the risk for tumors in the peripheral lung zones, where the majority of pulmonary adenocarcinomas arise. Furthermore, low-tar filter cigarettes may increase the risk for adenocarcinoma because of their higher nitrate content. The percentage of people smoking low-tar filter cigarettes in The Netherlands started to increase later than in the USA, but has steadily been increasing to 78% among male cigarette smokers and to 92% among female cigarette smokers in 1997. Younger people in The Netherlands were more inclined to smoke low-tar filter cigarettes than the elderly. The change in exposure to filter cigarettes has been less marked for women, because smoking became popular among women only since the 1960s. They mainly smoked low-tar filter cigarettes, and the proportion of adenocarcinoma remained considerably higher than for men during the whole study period.

The correlation between the effect of cigarette smoking on major histologic types of lung cancer has been evaluated in a meta-analysis by Khuder[14] based on studies identified through MEDLINE and CANCERLIT searches. A total of 48 studies published between 1970 and 1999 were identified. The combined estimates of relative risks (OR) for heaviest smoking intensity (30 or more cigarettes per day) ranged from 4.10 (95% confidence interval, CI, 3.16–5.31) for adenocarcinoma to 18.3 (95% CI 9.26–36.4) for small cell lung cancer (SCLC). The combined OR for longest duration of smoking (40 years or more) ranged from 3.80 (95% CI 2.35–6.16) for adenocarcinoma to 38.6 (95% CI 11.9–12.5) for SCLC. In women, the combined ORs for squamous cell carcinoma and SCLC were higher than those in men. The dose–response curve for intensity of smoking was steeper in women.

Finally, the histopathologic findings of lung carcinoma were evaluated in German uranium miners.[15] Two hundred and forty uranium miners with histologically or cytologically confirmed primary lung carcinoma were analyzed. The authors concluded that all cell types were associated with radon exposure, but high radiation exposure tended to increase the proportion of SCLC and squamous cell carcinoma, thus confirming the original observation by G Saccomanno and colleagues from the Colorado Plateau miners in the USA in the early 1970s.

REFERENCES

1. Franco J, Pérez-Hoyos S, Plaza P. Changes in lung-cancer mortality trends in Spain. *Int J Cancer* 2002; 97: 102–5.

2. Algranti E, Menezes AMB, Achutti AC. Lung cancer in Brazil. *Semin Oncol* 2001; 28: 143–52.

3. Trends in cigarette smoking among highschool students – United States, 1991–1999. *Morb Mort Wkly Rep* 2001; 15: 275–6.

4. Tønnesen P. How to reduce smoking among teenagers. *Eur Respir J* 2002; 19: 1–3.

5. Mannino DM, Ford E, Giovino GA, Thun M. Lung cancer mortality rates in birth cohorts in the United States from 1960–1994. *Lung Cancer* 2001; 31: 91–9.

6. Blizzard L, Dwyer T. Declining lung cancer mortality of young Australian women despite increased smoking is linked to reduced cigarette 'tar' yields. *Br J Cancer* 2001; 84: 392–6.

7. Blizzard L, Dwyer T. Lung cancer incidence in Australia: impact of filter-tip cigarettes with unchanged tar yields. *Int J Cancer* 2002; 97: 679–84.

8. Kreuzer M, Boffetta P, Whitley E et al. Gender differences in lung cancer risk by smoking: a multicentre case-control study in Germany and Italy. *Br J Cancer* 2000; 82: 227–33.

9. Siegfried JM. Women and lung cancer: Does oestrogen play a role? *Lancet Oncol* 2001; 2: 506–13.

10. Darby S, Whitley E, Doll R et al. Diet, smoking and lung cancer: a case–control study of 1000 cases and 1500 controls in South-West England. *Br J Cancer* 2001; 84: 728–35.

11. Kreuzer M, Gerken M, Kreienbrock L et al. Lung cancer in lifetime nonsmoking men – results of a case–control study in Germany. *Br J Cancer* 2001; 84: 134–40.

12. Janssen-Heijnen MLG, Goebergh J-WW. Trends in incidence and prognosis of the histological subtypes of lung cancer in North America, Australia, New Zealand and Europe. *Lung Cancer* 2001; 31: 123–37.

13. Jansen-Heijnen MLG, Coebergh J-WW, Klinkhamer PJJM et al. Is there a common etiology for the rising incidence of and decreasing survival with adenocarcinoma of the lung? *Epidemiology* 2001; 12: 256–8.

14. Khuder SA. Effect of cigarette smoking on major histological types of lung cancer: a meta-analysis. *Lung Cancer* 2001; 31: 139–48.

15. Kreuzer M, Müller KM, Brachner A et al. Histopathologic findings of lung carcinoma in German uranium miners. *Cancer* 2000; 89: 2613–21.

3
Prevention, early detection, and screening

Compared with 2001, new information from clinical trials on prevention has been scarce while the topic per se has been the subject of a couple of review articles,[1,2] including an overview of randomized lung cancer chemoprevention trials. Lippman and Spitz[2] conclude that all the definitive phase II and III lung cancer chemoprevention trials have produced negative (either neutral or harmful) primary endpoint results, whether in the primary, secondary or tertiary chemoprevention trial settings. These trials provided definitive answers to the questions they were designed to answer: lung cancer was not prevented by α-tocopherol, β-carotene, retinol, retinyl palmitate, N-acetylcysteine (NAC), or isotretinoin in smokers. They also provided provocative leads: isotretinoin may prevent lung cancer in never and former smokers, and α-tocopherol may even prevent lung cancer in smokers – probably at higher doses and longer durations than those tested in the present trials. A number of molecular targets such as retinoic acid (RA) receptors, aberrant methylation, p53, p16, and telomerase, are now being tested in the development of promising new drugs for chemoprevention of lung cancer.

Molecular targeting was discussed in a commentary by Pastorino[3] published in connection with a randomized US phase III trial of isotretinoin to prevent second primary tumors in patients with stage I non-small cell lung cancer (NSCLC).[4] In the latter study, 1166 patients with pathologic stage I NSCLC were included, 6 weeks to 3 years from definitive resection. None of them have received prior radio or chemotherapy. They were randomly assigned to receive a placebo or the retinoid isotretinoin (30 mg/day) for 3 years. Patients were stratified at randomization by tumor stage, histology, and smoking status. With a median follow-up of 3.5 years, there were no statistically significant differences between the placebo and isotretinoin arms with respect to the time to secondary primary tumors, recurrences, or mortality. A secondary multivariate and subset analysis suggested that isotretinoin was harmful in current smokers and beneficial in never smokers.[4]

With respect to early detection, much attention has been paid to the value of fluorescence bronchoscopy.[5,6] Hirsch et al[7] compared the ability of conventional white-light bronchoscopy (WBL) and laser-induced fluorescence endoscopic bronchoscopy (LIFE) to detect preneoplastic lung lesions in a randomized trial in which both the order of the procedures and the broncho-scopists were randomly assigned. The study included high-risk subjects with a 30 pack-year or more history of cigarette smoking, airflow obstruction, and either an abnormal sputum cytology (n = 48) or a previous or suspected lung cancer (n = 7). LIFE and WLB were performed on all patients. Biopsy speci-mens were assessed for histologic abnormalities, including the presence of angiogenic squamous dysplasia. A total of 391 biopsy specimens were taken from 55 patients. Thirty-two patients (58%; 95% confidence interval, CI, 44–71%) had at least one biopsy with moderate or severe dysplasia, and 19 (59%; 95% CI 41–76%) of these patients could be diagnosed solely upon the results of LIFE. LIFE was statistically significantly more sensitive than WLB for detecting moderate dysplasia or worse (68.8% versus 21.9%, respectively; dif-ference 46.9%; 95% CI 25–68%; p < 0.001). The relative sensitivities (WLB = 1.0) were 3.1 for LIFE and 3.7 for LIFE and WLB combined. The results were similar regardless of the order of the procedures or the order of the broncho-scopists. Also, LIFE was better at identifying angiogenic squamous dysplasia than WLB, indicating that the relative likelihood of getting a positive result in a sample with dysplasia compared with one without was 1.39 for LIFE (95% CI 1.17–1.65) versus a detection rate for WLB of 0.67 (95% CI 0.38–1.21). Altogether, the authors concluded that LIFE was more sensitive than WLB in detecting preneoplastic bronchial changes in high-risk subjects. The prognostic implication of this finding is not yet clear.

Kusunoki et al[8] presented their experience with detection of precancerous lesions and cancer, including carcinoma in situ (CIS), which are difficult to detect by WLB. Sixty-five patients with suspected lung cancer were examined by both methods, and biopsies were performed on 216 lesions. The accuracy of diagnosis of cancer and precancer by WLB was 48.6%, versus 72.7% by LIFE. The sensitivity of conventional bronchoscopy for detection of severe dysplasia or cancer was 61.2% and the specificity was 85.0%. With results by LIFE added, these values were 89.8% and 78.4%, respectively. Of nine patients with CIS only, LIFE showed one lesion, and only LIFE showed the extent of seven of the lesions. The autofluorescence of eight lesions was measured spectrofluorometrically; normal bronchial tissue, severe dysplasia, and cancer-ous tissue had spectral differences. The red/green intensity of cancers on his-tograms of LIFE images was generally greater than the ratios for metaplasia or normal bronchial wall. Evaluation of lesions by spectrofluorometry and digital signal intensity may make the results obtained with LIFE more objective. Kusunoki et al concluded that the use of both methods should facilitate early detection of preneoplasia. Semiautomated image cytometry has been applied to induced sputum as a screening procedure, but the validity of this method is still uncertain, and is awaiting large-scale feasibility studies.[9]

Other investigators, including Liloglou et al[10] and Ponticiello et al,[11] have found considerable cancer-specific genomic instability in bronchial lavage, which might be used as a potential marker for the early detection of lung cancer. Ponticiello et al[11] found evidence that $p53$ overexpression was present in bronchial dysplastic areas, and this may be a useful marker for identifying patients proceeding to squamous cell carcinoma and, in addition, may facilitate the detection of occult tumors.

Other features of preneoplastic lesions of the lung, including CD44 and CD44v6 expression, have been documented by Wimmel et al[12] as being altered on comparing normal and preneoplastic lesions. Also, reverse transcriptase polymerase chain reaction (RT–PCR) has been applied for the detection of cancer cells in sputum and peripheral blood using seven neuroendocrine marker transcripts including neural cell adhesion molecule (NCAM), PGP9.5, gastrin, gastrin receptor, synaptophysin, preprogastrin-releasing peptide (preproGRP), and GRP receptor.[13] Among these, preproGRP RT–PCR was the only assay with which illegitimate transcription in blood or sputum samples from healthy donors or patients with unrelated diseases did not interfere. However, it reproducibly detected up to 10 small cell lung cancer (SCLC) cells diluted in either 10 ml blood or 5 ml sputum samples. Single blood and sputum samples were collected directly before diagnostic bronchoscopy from 175 patients suspected to have lung cancer. Twenty-six of these had SCLC. Of these 26, 13 (50%) tested positive in the blood sample and 5 of 23 patients (22%) tested positive in the sputum sample. Moreover, among 92 patients with NSCLC, 25 (27%) had disseminated cancer cells in the peripheral blood. Further studies testing the usefulness of amplification of preproGRP transcripts from clinical samples are needed to evaluate whether this method is sufficiently sensitive and specific to detect disseminated or exfoliated lung cancer cells either in peripheral blood or in sputum samples.

In the case of detection of early superficial bronchogenic carcinoma (ESBC), the therapeutic option has until recently been surgical resection, but more conservative therapies, such as endoscopic therapies with photodynamic therapy, have been tested, and cryotherapy has also been proposed. Deygas et al[14] reported on the efficacy of cryotherapy through a rigid bronchoscope in patients with ESBC. Thirty-five patients were included, and multiple locations of ESBC were observed in 7. The complete response rates at both 1 month and 1 year were 91%. No severe adverse effects were noted. Local recurrence was observed within 4 years in 10 patients (28%). A follow-up period of at least 4 years was available in 22 patients; of these, 11 (50%) were long-term survivors. Deygas et al concluded that cryotherapy is an effective method of treatment in patients with ESBC. Owing to its relative tolerability compared with surgery, cryotherapy could be proposed as a first-line therapy in this population with carcinogenic risk. Obtaining information on this will depend on carefully performed systematic randomized trials with long-term follow-up, as reported by Thurer[15] in a commentary on the paper by Deygas et al.

The debate over the last couple of years about the potential value of screening for lung cancer has been continued in 2002, as evidenced by several review articles from both the USA and Europe, a consensus statement from the American Society of Thoracic Radiology, and an article also dealing with the economic implications of screening for lung cancer.[16–24] The various opinions are clearly expressed in two review articles, one by Patz et al[25] entitled 'CT screening for lung cancer: not ready for routine practice' and the other by Miettinen et al[26] entitled 'CT screening for lung cancer: coping with nihilistic recommendations'.

One major objection to screening is that it may unearth biologically unimportant tumors. Lung cancer is aggressive, but it is possible that tumors exist that do not manifest themselves during a life cut short by another smoking-related disease such as respiratory failure.[27] Another objection involves practicalities. Even with experienced operators, spiral computed tomography (CT) misses perihilar, peripheral, and lung cancers many of which can be clearly seen in retrospect. However, outcome might still be improved across the population where nodules are missed. A further question is whether screening might encourage complacency among smokers, and be regarded as a safety net to catch and cure those unlucky enough to develop lung cancer as a consequence of their smoking.

Large randomized trials to shed light on these major questions either have been implemented or are planned, both in North America and Europe. In the meantime, some data are emerging, mainly from Japan but also from the Early Lung Cancer Action Project (ELCAP) in New York. Using a mobile low-dose spiral CT scanner, Sone et al,[28] in a population of 5483 patients aged 40–74 years, using initial CT scans followed by repeat annual scans, detected nearly 11 times the expected annual number of early lung cancers. Henschke et al[29] reported the initial findings on repeat screening from the ELCAP group. A cohort of 1000 high-risk individuals was recruited for baseline and annual repeat CT screening. Of these, the test result was positive for a non-calcified nodule in 30 (2.5%). In 2 of these 30 cases, the individual died of an unrelated cause before diagnostic workup, and the nodules resolved in another 12 individuals. In the remaining 16 individuals, the absence of further growth was documented by repeat CT in 8 individuals, and further growth was documented in the remaining 8 individuals. All 8 individuals with further nodular growth underwent biopsy; malignancy was diagnosed in 7, including 6 with NSCLC, 5 of whom were stage IA and 1 of whom was stage IIIA, and the 1 SCLC was found to be of limited stage. The median size of these malignancies was 8 mm. In another two subjects, symptoms prompted an interim diagnosis of lung carcinoma. Neither of these malignancies was nodule-associated, but they were both endobronchial: one was a stage IIB NSCLC and the other was an SCLC of limited stage. Henschke et al concluded that false-positive screening test results are uncommon and usually manageable without biopsy. Compared with no screening, such screenings permit diagnosis at substantially earlier and thus more curable stages. Annual repetition of CT screening is sufficient to minimize symptom-prompted interim diagnoses of nodule-associated malignancies.

Tsukada et al[30] conducted a case–control study in which chest X-ray examinations for all participants and sputum cytology for high-risk participants were offered annually. Case subjects, who had died from lung cancer (174) and control subjects matched by sex, year of birth, residence, and smoking status, who had been alive at the time of diagnosis of the corresponding case, were selected from National Health Insurance holders. Screening histories of the subjects were compared between cases and matched controls for the identical calendar period before the time of diagnosis of the cases. The odds ratio of death from lung cancer for those screened within 12 months versus those not screened was 0.401, with adjustment by smoking index. These results suggest that annual lung cancer screening might reduce mortality from lung cancer by approximately 60%.

Another mass-screening program from Japan, conducted since 1982, used miniature chest X-ray for all screenees and sputum cytology for those with a smoking index of 600 or more (the smoking index is the average number of cigarettes smoked per day multiplied by the number of years of regular smoking – a smoking index of 600 is equivalent to 30 pack-years.[31] Within the 12 months before diagnosis, 241 of 328 cases (73.5%) had attended screening, compared with 1557 of 1886 controls (82.6%). The authors concluded that the mass screening program for lung cancer in Miyagi Prefecture was capable of reducing by 46% the risk of death from carcinoma of the lung.

REFERENCES

1. Goodman GE. Prevention of lung cancer. *Crit Rev Oncol Hematol* 2000; 33: 187–97.

2. Lippman SM, Spitz MR. Lung cancer chemoprevention: an integrated approach. *J Clin Oncol* 2001; 19(Suppl): 74s–82s.

3. Pastorino U. Molecular targeting: the new challenge in lung cancer prevention. *J Natl Cancer Inst* 2001; 93: 1190–1.

4. Lippman SM, Lee JJ, Karp DD et al. Randomized phase III intergroup trial of isotretinoin to prevent second primary tumors in stage I non-small-cell lung cancer. *J Natl Cancer Inst* 2001; 93: 605–18.

5. Hirsch FR, Franklin WA, Gazdar AF, Bunn PA Jr. Early detection of lung cancer: clinical perspectives of recent advances in biology and radiology. *Clin Cancer Res* 2001; 7: 5–21.

6. Kennedy TC, Lam S, Hirsch FR. Review of recent advances in fluorescence bronchoscopy in early localization of central airway lung cancer. *Oncologist* 2001; 6: 257–62.

7. Hirsch FR, Prindiville SA, Miller YE et al. Fluorescence versus white-light bronchoscopy for detection of preneoplastic lesions: a randomized study. *J Natl Cancer Inst* 2001; 93: 1385–91.

8. Kusunoki Y, Imamura F, Uda H et al. Early detection of lung cancer with laser-induced fluorescence endoscopy and spectrofluorometry. *Chest* 2000; 118: 1776–82.

9. Marek W, Kotschy-Lang N, Muti A et al. Can semi-automated image cytometry on induced sputum become a screening tool for lung cancer? *Eur Respir J* 2001; 18: 942–50.

10. Liloglou T, Maloney P, Zinarianos G et al. Cancer-specific genomic instability in bronchial lavage: a molecular tool for lung cancer detection. *Cancer Res* 2001; 61: 1624–8.

11. Ponticiello A, Barra E, Guiani U et al. p53 immunohistochemistry can identify bronchial dysplastic lesions proceeding to lung cancer: a prospective study. *Eur Respir J* 2000; 15: 547–52.

12. Wimmel A, Kogan E, Ramaswamy A, Schuermann M. Variant expression of CD44 in preneoplastic lesions of the lung. *Cancer* 2001; **92**: 1231–6.

13. Lacroix J, Becker HD, Woerner SM et al. Sensitive detection of rare cancer cells in sputum and peripheral blood samples of patients with lung cancer by preproGRP-specific RT–PCR. *Int J Cancer* 2001; **92**: 1–8.

14. Deygas N, Froudarakis M, Ozenne G, Vergnon J-M. Cryotherapy in early superficial bronchogenic carcinoma. *Chest* 2001; **120**: 26–31.

15. Thurer RJ. Cryotherapy in early lung cancer. *Chest* 2001: **120**: 3–5.

16. Ellis JRC, Gleeson FV. Lung cancer screening. *Br J Radiol* 2001; **74**: 478–85.

17. Marcus PM. Lung cancer screening: an update. *J Clin Oncol* 2001; **19**: 83s–6s.

18. Gorlova OY, Kimmel M, Henschke C. Modeling of long-term screening for lung carcinoma. *Cancer* 2001; **92**: 1531–40.

19. Grannis FW. Lung cancer overdiagnosis bias. *Chest* 2001; **119**: 322–3.

20. Prasson J, Arroligo AC. Spiral CT for lung cancer screening: Is it ready for prime time? *Cleveland Clin J Med* 2001; **68**: 74–81.

21. Aberle DR, Gamsu G, Henschke CI et al. A consensus statement of the Society of Thoracic Radiology. Screening for lung cancer with helical computed tomography. *J Thoracic Imag* 2001; **16**: 65–8.

22. Altorki N, Kent M, Pasmantier M. Detection of early-stage lung cancer: computed tomographic scan or chest radiograph? *J Thorac Cardiovasc Surg* 2001; **121**: 1053–7.

23. van Klaveren RJ, Habbema JDF, Pedersen JH et al. Lung cancer screening by low-dose spiral computed tomography. *Eur Respir J* 2001; **18**: 857–66.

24. Marchall D, Simpson KN, Earle CC, Chu C-W. Economic decision analysis model of screening for lung cancer. *Eur J Cancer* 2001; **37**: 1759–67.

25. Patz EF, Black WC, Goodman PC. CT screening for lung cancer: not ready for routine practice. *Radiology* 2001; **221**: 587–91.

26. Miettinen OS, Henschke CI. CT screening for lung cancer: coping with nihilistic recommendations. *Radiology* 2001; **221**: 592–6.

27. Anon. Opinion swings in favour of lung cancer screening. *Eur J Cancer* 2001; **37**: 1805–9.

28. Sone S, Li F, Yang Z-G et al. Results of three-year mass screening programme for lung cancer using mobile low-dose spiral computed tomography scanner. *Br J Cancer* 2001; **84**: 25–32.

29. Henschke CI, Naidich DP, Yankelevitz DF et al. Early Lung Cancer Action Project. Initial findings on repeat screening. *Cancer* 2001; **92**: 153–9.

30. Tsukada H, Kurita Y, Yokoyama A et al. An evaluation of screening for lung cancer in Niigata Prefecture, Japan: a population-based case–control study. *Br J Cancer* 2001; **85**: 1326–31.

31. Sagawa M, Tsubono Y, Saito Y et al. A case–control study for evaluating the efficacy of mass screening program for lung cancer in Miyagi Prefecture, Japan. *Cancer* 2001; **92**: 588–94.

4
Histopathology

In the chapter on histopathology in last year's *Annual*, the 1999 histologic classification of malignant epithelial tumors was presented, as published by the World Health Organization (WHO), based on recommendations by the Pathology Panel of the International Association for the Study of Lung Cancer (IASLC). The classification is listed in Table 4.1 and contains the morphologic codes of the International Classification of Diseases for

Table 4.1   Histologic classification of malignant lung and pleural tumours[a]

1 Epithelial tumours			
1.3 *Malignant*			
1.3.1 Squamous cell carcinoma			8070/3
Variants:			
1.3.1.1	Papillary		8052/3
1.3.1.2	Clear cell		8084/3
1.3.1.3	Small cell		8073/3
1.3.1.4	Basaloid		8083/3
1.3.2 Small cell carcinoma			8041/3
Variant:			
1.3.2.1	Combined		8045/3
1.3.3 Adenocarcinoma			8140/3
1.3.3.1	Acinar		8550/3
1.3.3.2	Papillary		8260/3
1.3.3.3	Bronchioloalveolar carcinoma		8250/3
	1.3.3.3.1	Non-mucinous	8252/3
	1.3.3.3.2	Mucinous	8253/3
	1.3.3.3.3	Mixed mucinous and non-mucinous or intermediate cell type	8254/3
1.3.3.4	Solid adenocarcinoma with mucin		8230/3
1.3.3.5	Adenocarcinoma with mixed subtypes		8255/3
1.3.3.6	Variants:		
	1.3.3.6.1	Well-differentiated fetal adenocarcinoma	8333/3
	1.3.3.6.2	Mucinous ('colloid') adenocarcinoma	8480/3
	1.3.3.6.3	Mucinous cystadenocarcinoma	8470/3
	1.3.3.6.4	Signet-ring adenocarcinoma	8490/3
	1.3.3.6.5	Clear cell adenocarcinoma	8310/3

Table 4.1	Continued		
1.3.4	Large cell carcinoma		8012/3
	Variants:		
	1.3.4.1	Large cell neuroendocrine carcinoma	8013/3
		1.3.4.1.1 Combined large cell neuroendocrine carcinoma	
	1.3.4.2	Basaloid carcinoma	8123/3
	1.3.4.3	Lymphoepithelioma-like carcinoma	8082/3
	1.3.4.4	Clear cell carcinoma	8310/3
	1.3.4.5	Large cell carcinoma with rhabdoid phenotype	8014/3
1.3.5	Adenosquamous carcinoma		8560/3
1.3.6	Carcinomas with pleomorphic, sarcomatoid, or sarcomatous elements		
	1.3.6.1	Carcinomas with spindle and/or giant cells	8030/3
		1.3.6.1.1 Pleomorphic carcinoma	8022/3
		1.3.6.1.2 Spindle cell carcinoma	8032/3
		1.3.6.1.3 Giant cell carcinoma	8031/3
	1.3.6.2	Carcinosarcoma	8980/3
	1.3.6.3	Pulmonary blastoma	8972/3
	1.3.6.4	Others	
1.3.7	Carcinoid tumour		8240/3
	1.3.7.1	Typical carcinoid	8240/3
	1.3.7.2	Atypical carcinoid	8249/3
1.3.8	Carcinomas of salivary gland type		
	1.3.8.1	Mucoepidermoid carcinoma	8430/3
	1.3.8.2	Adenoid cystic carcinoma	8200/3
	1.3.8.3	Others	
1.3.9	Unclassified carcinoma		8010/3

[a] Modified from Travis WD, Colby TV, Corrin B et al (eds). Histological typing of lung and pleural tumours. In: *WHO International Histological Classification of Tumours*, 3rd edn. Berlin: Springer-Verlag, 1999.

Oncology (ICD-O) and the Systemized Nomenclature of Medicine (SNOMED).[1] A summary of the new WHO classification of lung tumors was also published in 2001.[2]

A major change from the 1981 classification was the introduction of the concept of neuroendocrine tumors of the lung, which has been refined by the recognition of large neuroendocrine carcinomas and modifications of the criteria for atypical carcinoids. Neuroendocrine tumors are defined as the distinct subset of tumours that share certain morphologic, ultrastructural, and immunohistochemical characteristics. The major categories of morphologically identifiable neuroendocrine tumors are small cell carcinoma (SCLC), large cell neuroendocrine carcinoma, typical carcinoids, and atypical carcinoids. The criteria for a diagnosis of these tumors are given in Table 4.2.

Additional information concerning this group of tumors was published by Lyoda et al,[3] who analyzed 119 cases of large cell carcinoma from a total of 2070 primary lung carcinoma cases resected surgically between 1969 and

Table 4.2   Criteria for diagnosis of neuroendocrine tumors[a]

Tumor	Description[b]
Typical carcinoid	A tumor with carcinoid morphology and <2 mitoses per 2 mm^2 (10 HPF), lacking necrosis, and 0.5 cm or larger
Atypical carcinoid	A tumor with carcinoid morphology with 2–10 mitoses per 2 mm^2 (10 HPF) or necrosis (often punctate)
Large cell neuroendocrine carcinoma	1. A tumor with an NE morphology (organoid nesting, palisading, rosettes, trabeculae) 2. High mitotic rate: ≥ 11 per 2 mm^2 (10 HPF), median of 70 per 2 mm^2 (10 HPF) 3. Necrosis, often in large zones 4. Cytologic features of an NSCLC: large cell size, low nuclear-to-cytoplasmic ratio, vesicular or fine chromatin, and/or frequent nucleoli. Some tumors have fine nuclear chromatin and lack nucleoli, but qualify as NSCLC because of large cell size and abundant cytoplasm 5. Positive immunohistochemical staining for one or more NE markers (other than NSE) and/or NE granules by electron microscopy
Small cell carcinoma	1. Small size (generally less than the diameter of three small resting lymphocytes) 2. Scant cytoplasm 3. Nuclei: finely granular nuclear chromatin, absent or faint nucleoli 4. High mitotic rate (≥ 11 per 2 mm^2) (10 HPF), median of 80 per 2 mm^2 (10 HPF) 5. Frequent necrosis, often in large zones

[a] From Travis WD, Colby TV, Corrin B et al (eds). Histological typing of lung and pleural tumours. In: *WHO International Histological Classification of Tumours*. Berlin: Springer-Verlag, 1999.
[b] For an explanation of HPF (high-power field) area and mitosis counting, see Travis et al, p. 10. NE, neuroendocrine; NSCLC, non-small cell lung cancer; NSE, neuron-specific enolase.

1990. Using light microscopy, electron microscopy, and immunohistochemical staining, they reclassified these cases into large cell neuroendocrine carcinoma (LCNEC), large cell carcinoma with neuroendocrine differentiation (LCCND), large cell carcinoma with neuroendocrine morphology (LCCNM), and classic large cell carcinoma (CLCC). Multivariate analysis showed that large cell carcinomas with neuroendocrine features, which combine LCNEC, LCCND, and LCCNM, have an impact on both the overall survival and disease-free survival of patients. The clinical behavior of LCCNM was similar to that of LCNEC. The results of multivariate analysis for overall survival and disease-free survival comparing large cell carcinomas with neuroendocrine features versus CLCC are given in Table 4.3. In addition, the proportion of cases with elevated lactate dehydrogenase (LDH) was significantly higher for large cell carcinomas with neuroendocrine features than for those without, while the proportion of cases with elevated neuron-specific enolase (NSE) was not significantly different among the four categories. Lyoda et al concluded that large cell carcinomas with neuroendocrine features appear to be more clinically aggressive than CLCC without neuroendocrine features and that these findings may have an impact on therapeutic strategies.

Also, subgroups of neuroendocrine tumors designated 'typical' and 'atypical' pulmonary carcinoids have been subjected to detailed analysis. A computerized search of the medical records for pulmonary carcinoid tumors at the Mayo Clinic in the USA from 1976 to 1997 revealed 517 patients, of whom 36 were identified with pulmonary carcinoid tumors involving regional thoracic lymph nodes but without distant metastases.[4] All histologic specimens were reexamined using the current WHO criteria for classifying pulmonary neuroendocrine

Table 4.3   Overall and disease-free survivals for each histologic type of tumor

Overall survival Tumor[a]	Median survival time (months)	5-year survival rate	95% confidence interval
CLCC	25	0.484	0.319–0.649
Large cell carcinoma with neuroendocrine features	16.5	0.323	0.205–0.441
LCNEC	19	0.353	0.208–0.498
LCCND	8	0.222	0–0.494
LCCNM	14	0.273	0.010–0.545

Disease-free survival Tumor[a]	Median survival time (months)	5-year survival rate	95% confidence interval
CLCC			
Large cell carcinoma with neuroendocrine features	24	0.433	0.278–0.588
LCNEC	11.5	0.254	0.148–0.360
LCCND	12.5	0.274	0.143–0.405
LCCNM	6	0.222	0–0.494

[a] CLCC, classic large cell carcinoma; LCNEC, large cell neuroendocrine carcinoma; LCCND, large cell carcinoma with neuroendocrine differentiation; LCCNM, large cell carcinoma with neuroendocrine morphology.

tumors. Twenty-three patients had typical carcinoid tumors with thoracic lymph node involvement, and at the last follow-up, 19 patients had no evidence of disease, 2 had developed systemic metastases and are still alive, and 2 had died. Eleven patients had atypical carcinoid tumors with thoracic lymph node involvement. At the last follow-up, 4 patients had no evidence of disease, 7 had developed systemic metastases within a median time of 17 months, and 6 with systemic metastases died shortly thereafter (median survival time 25.5 months), while 1 is still alive. Two patients had been reclassified with large cell neuroendocrine carcinoma at the time of review. Both of these patients had developed systemic metastases at 4 months and 21 months after diagnosis, and had died at 15 months and 21 months after diagnosis, respectively. The data suggest that patients with atypical pulmonary carcinoid tumors with regional lymph node metastases have a high likelihood of developing recurrent disease if treated with surgical resection alone, and have significantly worse outcome compared with patients who have typical carcinoid tumors with thoracic lymph node involvement.

At the Mayo Clinic, two sets of first-degree relatives diagnosed with primary pulmonary carcinoid tumors with no clinical features of multiple endocrine neoplasia type 1 (MEN1) were identified in a pair of siblings and in a mother and daughter.[5] Mutations in the MEN1 gene were sought using polymerase chain reaction (PCR) analysis on paraffin-embedded tissue from two members of one of the families. None of these patients and no family members had features of MEN1. DNA analysis did not detect germline mutations in the MEN1 gene. The findings suggested a novel, rare germline mutation specific to the development of pulmonary carcinoids. With respect to pulmonary carcinoids, the charactericistic features and outcome have been subjected to a retrospective analysis of 142 patients from four major hospitals in Israel. The results of this study are similar to reports from major oncology centers outside Israel.[6]

The prognosis of rarer subtypes of bronchogenic carcinoma has been subjected to retrospective study. Breathnach et al[7] studied patients with stage I bronchioloalveolar carcinoma or adenocarcinoma other than bronchioloalveolar carcinoma resected between 1984 and 1992 at the Harvard Medical School. A total of 138 patients were identified. Thirty-three had bronchioloalveolar carcinoma and 105 patients had adenocarcinoma. Eleven (33%) of the patients with bronchioloalveolar carcinoma had never smoked cigarettes, versus 9 (9%) of the patients with adenocarcinoma ($p = 0.0036$). There were no significant differences between patients with bronchioloalveolar carcinoma and adenocarcinoma in sex distribution and overall recurrence rate. Of the 12 patients with recurrent bronchioloalveolar carcinoma, 1 (8%) had extrathoracic disease develop at the site of the first recurrence, compared with 49% of the patients with recurrent adenocarcinoma ($p < 0.001$). The 5-year survival rates in patients with bronchioloalveolar carcinoma and in those with adenocarcinoma were 83% and 63%, respectively ($p = 0.04$). Stage I bronchioloalveolar carcinoma is thus more likely to occur in non-smokers, and survival is longer in patients with this subtype than in patients with other carcinomas.

REFERENCES

1. Travis WD, Colby TV, Corrin B et al (eds). Histological typing of lung and pleural tumours. In: *WHO International Histological Classification of Tumours*, 3rd edn. Berlin: Springer-Verlag, 1999.

2. Brambilla E, Travis WD, Colby TV et al. The new World Health Organization classification of lung tumours. *Eur Respir J* 2001; **18**: 1059–68.

3. Lyoda A, Hiroshima K, Toyozaki T et al. Clinical characterization of pulmonary large cell neuroendocrine carcinoma and large cell carcinoma with neuroendocrine morphology. *Cancer* 2001; **91**: 1992–2000.

4. Thomas CF Jr, Tazelaar HD, Jett JR. Typical and atypical pulmonary carcinoids. Outcome in patients presenting with regional lymph node involvement. *Chest* 2001; **119**: 1143–50.

5. Oliveira AM, Tazelaar HD, Wentzlaff KA et al. Familial pulmonary carcinoid tumors. *Cancer* 2001; **91**: 2104–9.

6. Fink G, Krelbaum T, Yellin A et al. Pulmonary carcinoid. Presentation, diagnosis, and outcome in 142 cases in Israel and review of 640 cases from the literature. *Chest* 2001; **119**: 1647–51.

7. Breathnach OS, Kwiatkowsky DJ, Finkelstein DM et al. Bronchioloalveolar carcinoma of the lung: recurrences and survival in patients with stage I disease. *J Thorac Cardiovasc Surg* 2001; **121**: 42–7.

5
Staging, staging procedures, and prognostic factors

Clinical staging of lung cancer helps to determine the extent of disease and stratify patients into similar prognostic and therapeutic categories. For lung cancer patients, an important goal is to separate those with potential resectable disease from those who are unresectable. The most recent staging system for lung cancer was published in 1997 (Table 5.1; Figures 5.1–5.5), replacing the 1986 classification.

Evaluation of the International Staging System for Lung Cancer has been performed in Italian, Dutch, and Polish studies, as discussed in last year's *Annual*. In 2001, the 1997 TNM staging system was evaluated by the Japanese based on 3043 lung cancer patients who underwent pulmonary resection at the National Cancer Center Hospital, Tokyo.[1] The 5-year survival rate showed

Table 5.1	Revised (1997) TNM stage classification for lung cancer[a,b]
Stage	**TNM classification**
Occult	TXN0M0
0	TisNOMO
IA	TIN0M0
IB	T2N0M0
IIA	T12N1M0
IIB	T2N1M0 T3N0M0
IIIA	T3N1M0, T1N2M0, T2N2M0, T3N2M0
IIIB	T4(any N)M0, (any T)N3M0
IV	(any T) (any N)M1

[a] Adapted from Mountain CF. Revisions in the International System for Staging Lung Cancer. *Chest* 1997; 111: 1710–17.
[b] Satellite tumor nodule(s) in ipsilateral primary tumor lobe(s) is designated T4. Separate tumor nodule(s) in ipsilateral non-primary tumor lobe(s) is designated M1.

Stage I
No lymph node involvement

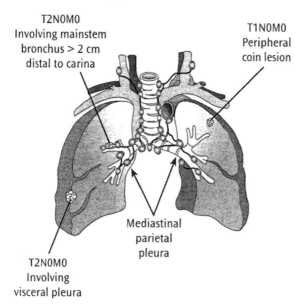

T2N0M0
Involving mainstem
bronchus > 2 cm
distal to carina

T1N0M0
Peripheral
coin lesion

Mediastinal
parietal
pleura

T2N0M0
Involving
visceral pleura

Figure 5.1

Stage I disease.
(Reproduced, with
permission, from
Mountain CF. A new
international staging
system for lung cancers.
Chest 1986; **89:**
225S–33S.)

Stage IIA
Intrapulmonary and/or hilar nodes involved
Tumor < 3 cm

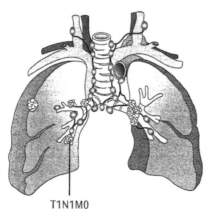

T1N1M0
< 3 cm involving
ipsilateral peribronchial and/or
ipsilateral hilar lymph nodes

Figure 5.2

Stage IIA disease. (Adapted, with
permission, from Mountain CF. A new
international staging system for lung
cancers. *Chest* 1986; **89:** 225S–33S.)

Stage IIB

Intrapulmonary and/or hilar nodes involved

Tumor > 3 cm

T2N1M0 or T3N0M0
Involving visceral pleura
and peribronchial and
hilar lymph nodes

Involving main
bronchus
and hilar
lymph nodes

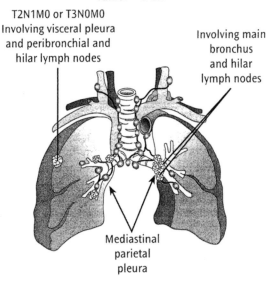

Mediastinal
parietal
pleura

Figure 5.3

Stage IIB. (Adapted, with permission, from Mountain CF. A new international staging system for lung cancers. *Chest* 1986; **89:** 225S–33S.)

Stage IIIA

T3N1M0
Peripheral tumor
involving chest wall
and intrapulmonary
lymph nodes

T2N2M0
> 3 cm tumor
involving ipsilateral
hilar and
mediastinal
lymph nodes

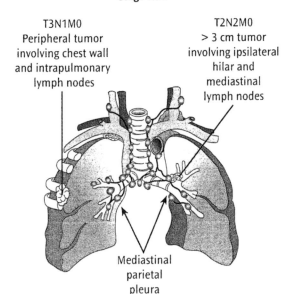

Mediastinal
parietal
pleura

Figure 5.4

Stage IIIA disease. (Adapted, with permission, from Mountain CF. A new international staging system for lung cancers. *Chest* 1986; **89:** 225S–33S.)

Stage IIIB

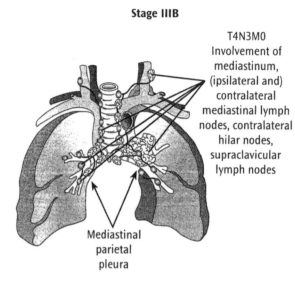

T4N3M0
Involvement of
mediastinum,
(ipsilateral and)
contralateral
mediastinal lymph
nodes, contralateral
hilar nodes,
supraclavicular
lymph nodes

Mediastinal
parietal
pleura

Figure 5.5

Stage IIIB disease.
(Reproduced, with
permission, from
Mountain CF. A new
international staging
system for lung cancers.
Chest 1986; **89:**
225S–33S.)

no significant difference between stages IB and IIA, between stages IIA and IIB, or between stages IIIB and IV. The results are thus in concurrence with the data from the Dutch study showing no survival difference between stages IB and IIA, and also a considerable heterogeneity for patients included in stage III. In a commentary on the article by Naruke et al, Putnam[2] concluded that the current staging system is in transition – both anatomically and biologically. Further refinements in anatomic staging will require much larger populations to detect smaller survival differences. Furthermore, the exclusive use of cStage and pStage anatomic characteristics will gradually decline as molecular staging evolves. This evaluation will mark 'the end of the beginning' of anatomic lung cancer staging.[2]

NON-SMALL CELL LUNG CANCER

Similar considerations to the above were expressed by Cox et al[3] based on a retrospective analysis of 167 patients with resected stage I–IIIA non-small cell lung cancer (NSCLC). The authors conclude that angiogenesis, epidermal growth factor receptor (EGFR) and matrix metalloproteinase-9 (MMP-9) expression all provide prognostic information independent of TNM stage, allowing a more accurate outcome prediction for the individual patient. Also, Mott et al[4] have called for a stage revision based on an analysis of patients with NSCLC with and without pleural effusion.

Fortunately, the International Association for the Study of Lung Cancer (IASLC) has recently established a Staging Committee, the purpose of which is to scrutinize the present staging system based on data from cooperative groups from North America, Europe, and Japan, with the aim of establishing a new system that is more optimal.

With respect to staging, chest radiography and computed tomography (CT) scanning are the conventional imaging procedures, and have more recently been complemented by positron emission tomography (PET) with [18F]fluorodeoxyglucose (FDG). The invasive procedures have included bronchoscopy, mediastinoscopy, transbronchial needle aspiration, and transthoracic needle aspiration.

For staging of the mediastinum of patients with known NSCLC, Esnaola et al[5] used a decision-analytic model to compare the health outcomes and cost-effectiveness of three staging strategies: (i) chest CT alone, (ii) selective mediastinoscopy, and (iii) routine mediastinoscopy. The estimates of the sensitivity and specificity of CT and mediastinoscopy were obtained from a published meta-analysis and from several prospective studies, respectively. The overall effectiveness and cost of each strategy were functions of the proportion of patients accurately staged and of the risks, benefits, and costs of the diagnostic tests and treatments used. Esnaola et al adopted a societal perspective and calculated incremental cost-effectiveness ratios (ICERs) as cost per quality-adjusted life-year (QALY) gained. They concluded that routine mediastinoscopy maximizes quality-adjusted life expectancy in patients with known NSCLC, and its ICER compares favorably with those of other currently accepted medical technologies. The survival benefit and cost-effectiveness of this strategy are greater in patients with T2 and T3 tumors, and are likely to improve with advances in multimodal therapy.

With respect to chest radiography versus CT scan, Altorki et al.[6] performed a retrospective study comparing two groups of patients with biopsy-proven NSCLC. In the first group of 32 patients, the tumors were detected by a CT scan. In a second group ($n = 101$), the lung cancers were detected on routine chest X-ray films. Patients with pulmonary symptoms or a history of cancer were excluded. A significantly greater number of patients undergoing CT scan had stage IA disease compared with those having an X-ray film. Of the 32 patients in the group having a scan, 10 had tumors 1 cm or less in size, versus 6 of 101 in the group having a chest radiograph. Additionally, there was a significant reduction in advanced-stage disease in the group having a scan.

As to invasive procedures, Herth et al[7] developed a new method of endobronchial ultrasonography (EBUS) as an adjunct to conventional bronchoscopy. They describe their experience of the assessment of EBUS in 648 patients, who also underwent bronchoscopy. The mean procedure time for the bronchoscopies was 18.9 minutes, while the mean time for EBUS was 6.3 minutes. Side-effects were comparatively rare. Herth et al concluded that the method extends the endoscopist's view beyond the tracheobronchial wall, and might add even to radiologic diagnostic procedures such as CT and PET scans in that regard, but unfortunately no data are given on the sensitivity and specificity of the procedure.

The staging of the mediastinum in NSCLC by mediastinoscopy suffers from a low sensitivity, leading to a number of patients with unforeseen N2 disease at thoracotomy. For this reason, Oosterhuis et al[8] initiated a study to assess whether preoperative staging could be improved by serial sectioning and immunohistochemical staining of mediastinoscopy biopsies. In 183 consecutive patients with NSCLC, a thoracotomy was performed after a thorough mediastinal staging by CT scan and cervical mediastinoscopy. In 158 patients (88%), a mediastinal node dissection was performed, revealing unforeseen N2 disease in 24 cases (15%). The preserved mediastinoscopy biopsies of these patients were retrospectively serially sectioned and stained with an anti-keratin monoclonal antibody (MNF 116). Metastases could be identified in seven cases (30%), reducing unforeseen N2 disease from 15% to 10%. The number of patients who could theoretically benefit from neoadjuvant therapy would have been increased by at least 10%.

With regard to evaluation of the mediastinum with special focus on nuclear medicine imaging, a number of reviews have been published,[9–15] including one employing a systematic search in the MEDLINE and EMBASE databases and the Cochrane Controlled Trials Register.[16] The authors identified 55 original works on the diagnostic performance of FDG–PET in the investigation of NSCLC. For diagnosis of NSCLC, the mean sensitivities and specificities were, respectively, 0.96 (standard error, SE, 0.01) and 0.78 (SE 0.03) for dedicated PET, and 0.92 (SE 0.04) and 0.86 (SE 0.04) for gamma-camera PET. In the mediastinal staging of NSCLC, the results were 0.83 (SE 0.02) and 0.96 (SE 0.01) for dedicated PET and 0.81 (SE 0.04) and 0.95 (SE 0.02) for gamma-camera PET. The authors conclude that dedicated PET could be a valuable tool in the diagnosis and staging of NSCLC, but studies of populations with a lower prevalence of NSCLC are recommended.

FDG–PET has also been validated for differentiation of unknown pulmonary lesions. The results indicate that FDG–PET contributes efficiently to the detection of malignancy of tumors larger than 1 cm, but positive lymph node imaging must not preclude surgery, and requires histologic proof. Discrimination of benign and malignant pulmonary tumors by FDG–PET appears to be hampered in inflammatory lesions.[17] The latter issue is also elucidated in an article by Zhuang et al,[18] who suggest, based on in vitro studies and clinical studies employing a retrospective analysis of 76 patients who had dual-time FDG–PET scans, that dual-time imaging appears to be useful in distinguishing malignant from benign lesions. The need for further diagnostic procedures in patients with PET–FDG scans in order to avoid overstaging and allow better surgical patient selection has also been emphasized by Poncelet et al.[19]

The sensitivity, specificity, and accuracy of CT and PET for detecting metastatic lymphadenopathy have been analyzed in several studies,[20–23] including retrospective analyses performed on 77 and 196 patients, respectively, by Gupta et al.[20] and Lee et al.[21]

PET has been applied to patients who were candidates for curative-intent radiotherapy.[23,24] MacManus et al[24] prospectively studied 153 patients with unresectable NSCLC who were candidates for radical radiotherapy after conventional staging and had PET scans. Patients were allocated both 'pre-PET' and 'post-PET' stages. Subsequent management was recorded. Survival analysis was used to compare the validity of pre-PET and post-PET staging. After PET, 107 patients (70%) actually received radical therapies (radical radiotherapy with or without concurrent chemotherapy, $n = 102$; radical surgery, $n = 5$), while 46 patients (30%) received palliative treatment because of PET-detected distant metastasis ($n = 28$; 18%) or extensive locoregional disease ($n = 18$; 12%). Palliative therapies were radiotherapy ($n = 33$), chemotherapy ($n = 12$), and supportive care ($n = 1$). All five surgically treated patients underwent potentially curative resections after downstaging by PET. For radically treated patients, post-PET stage ($p = 0.0041$), but not pre-PET stage ($p = 0.19$), was strongly associated with survival. Radically treated patients survived longer than those treated palliatively ($p = 0.02$; 1-year survival rates 69% and 44%, respectively). MacManus et al concluded that PET-assisted staging detected unsuspected metastasis in 20%, strongly influenced choice of treatment strategy, frequently impacted radiotherapy planning, and was a powerful predictor of survival. The potential impact of FDG–PET is even greater in radical radiotherapy candidates with NSCLC than in surgical candidates.

Similar conclusions were reached by Mah et al[25] who recommended that FDG–PET data should be integrated into treatment planning of NSCLC, particularly for three-dimensional (3D) conformal techniques.

PET imaging has been conducted following surgical staging of NSCLC after induction therapy with chemotherapy, chemoradiation or radiation alone.[26] PET had a positive predictive value of 98% for detecting residual viable disease in the primary tumor in 56 patients, while it overstaged nodal status in 33% of patients, understaged nodal status in 15%, and was correct in 52%. PET correctly classified all patients with M1 disease. PET accurately detected residual viable primary tumor after induction therapy, but not the involvement of mediastinal lymph nodes.

Other techniques, such as mediastinoscopy, have been explored after induction chemotherapy in NSCLC. Mateu-Navarro et al[27] evaluated the technical feasibility and the sensitivity, specificity, and accuracy of remediastinoscopy in restaging 26 patients with N2 NSCLC receiving neoadjuvant chemotherapy. Twenty-four patients underwent remediastinoscopy, and in 12 remediastinoscopy was positive. The remaining 12 patients were operated on and the tumors resected: 5 pneumonectomies and 7 lobectomies. Lymphadenectomy specimens showed residual disease in mediastinal lymph nodes in 5 patients (pN2) and hilar lymph nodes in 1 patient (pN1). The other 6 patients were free of nodal disease, and 4 of them presented no lung involvement. The sensitivity, specificity, and accuracy of remediastinoscopy were 0.7, 1, and 0.8, respectively. Except for a surgical wound infection, no complications were encountered. Remediastinoscopy is a technically feasible staging tool with high diagnostic accuracy that may be useful in the selection of patients who can be served best by complete resection after neoadjuvant chemotherapy. Further studies on the role of remediastinoscopy are needed.

The optimal approach to the investigation of possible distant metastases in patients with apparently operable NSCLC who do not have symptoms suggesting metastatic disease remains controversial. The Canadian Lung Oncology Group[28] has shed further light on this issue by conducting a randomized, controlled trial recruiting 634 patients with apparently operable, suspected, or proven NSCLC without findings on history, physical examination, laboratory testing, or imaging suggesting extrathoracic metastases. Patients were randomly allocated to receive either mediastinoscopy and CT of the chest and then, depending on the results, immediate thoracotomy or bone scintigraphy and CT scanning of the head, liver and adrenal glands. The relative risk of thoracotomy without cure in the full-investigation group versus the limited-investigation group was 0.80 (95% confidence interval (CI) 0.56–1.13; $p = 0.20$). Forty-three patients in the full-investigation group and 61 patients in the limited-investigation group underwent a thoracotomy but subsequently had recurrence (relative risk 0.70; 95% CI 0.47–1.03; $p = 0.07$). Patients in the full-investigation group were more likely to have avoided thoracotomy because of extrathoracic metastatic disease than those in the limited-investigation group (22 patients versus 10 patients, respectively; relative risk 2.19; 95% CI 1.04–4.59; $p = 0.04$). Full investigation for metastatic disease in patients with NSCLC without symptoms or signs of metastatic disease may reduce the number of thoracotomies without cure. With the recent development and use of PET scanning in NSCLC, the approach to the proper and most efficient staging of NSCLC is rapidly changing, and large prospective trials, including cost-effectiveness analysis, are awaited with great interest by both clinicians and healthcare providers.

Spread to extrathoracic locations, such as the bone marrow, has been further evaluated in detail by Mattioli et al[29] and Poncelet et al.[30] The latter authors investigated the presence of occult bone marrow metastases using monoclonal primary antibodies directed against low-molecular-weight cytokeratins in 99 patients undergoing surgical treatment. The overall prevalence of occult micrometastasis was 22.2% (22 out of 99). The presence of occult bone marrow metastasis was not correlated with pathology or T status, nor was it a predictor of overall or disease-free survival. Data from this study are thus in contrast to those from previously published studies, with respect both to the prevalence of bone marrow micrometastatic cells and to its impact on prognosis. Based on a small study of 21 consecutive patients (18 NSCLC), Mattioli et al[29] suggested that the diagnosis of bone marrow isolated tumor cells has clinical relevance, and that the preoperative assessment should be performed by rib segment resection or methods other than iliac crest aspirate or biopsy. Among 18 patients with NSCLC, 7 of 10 with adenocarcinoma had cytokeratin-positive cells in the rib bone marrow, while only two of 8 with squamous cell cancer turned out to be positive. None of the serial sections obtained from the posterior iliac crest biopsies revealed the presence of isolated tumor cells or clusters either at morphologic or immunohistochemical evaluation. No survival data were reported. The utility of bone marrow evaluation in the staging of NSCLC remains unclear.

As mentioned above, the current staging of NSCLC is based on the TNM system, but data on molecular biological substaging are accumulating rapidly and several biological staging models have been suggested. In 2001, numerous articles were published providing prognostic information on a number of tumor markers, such as DNA content and S-phase fraction determined by flow cytometry,[31] p53,[32] chromosomal aberrations (including c-erb B-2),[33] p16 expression and telomerase activity,[34–36] vascular endothelial growth factor (VEGF) expression,[37] cell cycle regulators,[38] various proteases and adhesion molecules potentially involved in angiogenesis and metastasis,[39–44] proteins involved in the proliferation of tumor cells, such as minichromosome maintenance protein 2 (MCM2),[45] expression of nucleolar protein p120,[46] thioredoxin,[47] dihydrodiol dehydrogenase,[48] and polysialic acid,[49] and, finally, pretreatment serum levels of HER2/neu (c-ErbB-2) oncoprotein.[50] Other parameters, such as hypoxia inducible factor 1α and 2K coagulation tests, have also been evaluated and confirmed as predictors of survival, although not independently of other prognostic factors.[51,52]

Among clinical prognostic factors, performance status has been recognized as one of the most important. In a study by Ando et al,[53] accuracy in the assessment of performance status was evaluated by comparing results among patients, nurses, and oncologists. Two hundred and six patients with inoperable, advanced NSCLC were investigated prospectively. There was a significant difference among the assessments by the three groups ($p < 0.001$). Oncologists gave the healthiest performance status assessment, nurses an intermediate assessment, and patients the poorest. When included separately in the Cox model, the assessment by each group was significantly correlated with survival. However, assessment by patients themselves failed to distinguish survival of patients with performance status 1 or 2. The results indicate that assessment by patients themselves is different from those by nurses and oncologists.

Quality of life has also been identified as an important prognostic factor by interview of 129 lung cancer patients.[54] Quality of life was measured using the Nottingham Health Profile, the European Organization for Research and Treatment of Cancer Quality of Life Questionnaire (EORTC-QLQ) and its lung cancer supplementary questionnaire, in addition to a study-specific questionnaire collecting data on demographic, social, clinical, and performance status. Multivariate analyses showed that prediagnosis global quality of life was the most significant predictor of the length of survival, even after adjusting for known prognostic factors such as age, extent of disease, and global quality of life, while performance status, sex, and weight loss were not. The authors concluded that prediagnosis quality of life should be considered as a clinical status that has to be established by physicians before treatment starts, since it is such an important predictor of survival.

SMALL CELL LUNG CANCER

Rather than using the detected TNM staging system, small cell lung cancer (SCLC) is usually classified into two stages: limited disease (LD) and extensive disease (ED). However, the criteria for these two categories remain controversial. The widely used Veterans Administration Lung Study Group (VALG) definition of LD includes patients with primary tumor and nodal involvement limited to one hemithorax. In contrast, the IASLC recommends that LD should additionally include all patients without distant metastasis. According to the IASLC classification, only patients with distant metastasis – (any T) (any N) M1 – are considered as having extensive disease, i.e. the IASLC criteria include more patients in the prognostically superior LD category than the VALG definition. As a consequence, since treatment modalities for LD and ED could be different, individual clinical outcome of SCLC patients may be influenced by the staging system chosen. Micke et al[55] reviewed 109 consecutive SCLC patients from one institution in the period from 1989 to 1999 and classified them according to the two staging classifications, LD-VALG and ED-VALG or LD-IASLC and ED-IASLC, and LD–ED, which is the overlapping group. The prognosis of this overlapping group (LD–ED: median survival 291 days) was not statistically different from patients with limited disease defined by VALG criteria (LD-VALG: 385 days; $p = 0.42$). On the other hand, the survival difference between LD–ED patients and the ED-IASLC population was significant (ED-IASLC: 208 days; $p = 0.05$), indicating that LD–ED patients should rather be included in the LD category. This is further supported by the results of a multivariate Cox regression analysis with all clinically relevant data. Only stage as defined by IASLC criteria was an independent prognostic factor in the likelihood-ratio forward and backward model, confirming the greater discriminatory power of the IASLC definition. Micke et al concluded that the IASLC staging criteria for SCLC patients have a higher prognostic impact and are therefore preferable in clinical practice and future therapeutic trials. Further data based on larger databases are needed in order to confirm the above conclusions.

FDG–PET imaging has also been evaluated in patients with SCLC and compared with currently recommended staging procedures in two German studies by Hauber et al[56] and Schumacher et al.[57] Both studies are rather small, including 24 and 31 patients, respectively. In the study by Schumacher et al, identifical results from FDG–PET and the sum of other staging procedures were obtained in 23 of 36 examinations (6 had limited disease, 12 had extensive disease, and 5 had no evidence of disease). In contrast to the results of conventional staging, FDG–PET indicated extensive disease, resulting in an upstaging in 7 patients. It was concluded that FDG–PET has potential for use as a simplified staging tool for SCLC – a conclusion that is supported also by Hauber et al based on their experience where PET was mainly performed in patients with local regional SCLC. Investigations with a larger number of patients in a prospective study are needed to further elucidate the usefulness of this and other imaging procedures, such as technetium-99m methoxy-isobutylisonitrile (Tc-99m MIBI) chest imaging[58] in the staging of SCLC.

SCLC is derived from the neural ectoderm and often displays the neuro-endocrine features characteristic of amine precursor uptake and decarboxylation (APUD)-oma tumors. A number of tumor markers have been identified as prognostic markers for SCLC, including neuron-specific enolase (NSE), which has also been confirmed in a recent study by Giovanella et al,[59] who compared immunoradiometric assay of chromogranin A (CgA) with NSE in 64 cases of SCLC and in 102 cases of NSCLC and 106 cases of non-malignant lung diseases as controls. NSE reflected disease extent more accurately than CgA (U-test: CgA $p < 0.05$, NSE $p < 0.001$). The value of cerebrospinal fluid gastrin-releasing peptide (GRP) in the diagnosis of leptomeningeal metastases from SCLC has also been confirmed by Castro et al.[60] The value of lactate dehydrogenase (LDH) levels in SCLC was tested by Tas et al,[61] and in a multivariate analysis its value was reconfirmed as an important biochemical marker. Of the new biochemical markers, Micke et al.[62] found c-erbB-2 expression in more than 20% of SCLC examined and that this expression was an important prognostic factor for survival. The effect of c-erbB-2 expression seems to be more important in advanced stages of the disease than in limited disease.

REFERENCES

1. Naruke T, Tsuchiya R, Kondo H, Asamura H. Prognosis and survival after resection for bronchogenic carcinoma based on the 1997 TNM-staging classification: the Japanese experience. *Ann Thorac Surg* 2001; 71: 1759–64.

2. Putnam JB Jr. The anatomic basis for lung cancer staging: the end of the beginning? *Ann Thorac Surg* 2001; 71: 1757–8.

3. Cox G, Jones JL, Andi A et al. A biological staging model for operable non-small cell lung cancer. *Thorax* 2001; 56: 561–6.

4. Mott FE, Sharma N, Ashley P. Malignant pleural effusion in non-small cell lung cancer – time for a stage revision? *Chest* 2001; 119: 317–18.

5. Esnaola NF, Lazarides SN, Mentzer SJ, Kuntz KM. Outcomes and cost-effectiveness of alternative staging strategies for non-small-cell lung cancer. *J Clin Oncol* 2002; 20: 263–73.

6. Altorki N, Kent M, Pasmantier M. Detection of early-stage lung cancer: computed tomographic scan or chest radiograph? *J Thorac Cardiovasc Surg* 2001; 121: 1053–7.

7. Herth F, Becker HD, Manegold C, Drings P. Endobronchial ultrasound (EBUS) – assessment of a new diagnostic tool in bronchoscopy for staging of lung cancer. *Onkologie* 2001; 24: 151–4.

8. Oosterhuis JWA, Theunissen PHMH, Bollen ECM. Improved preoperative mediastinal staging in non-small-cell lung cancer by serial sectioning and immunohistochemical staining of lymph-node biopsies. *Eur J Cardio-Thorac Surg* 2001; 20: 335–8.

9. Salminen E, MacManus M. Impact of FDG-labelled positron emission tomography imaging on the management of non-small-cell lung cancer. *Ann Med* 2001; 33: 404–9.

10. Pieterman RM, van Putten JWG, Meuzelaar JJ et al. Preoperative

staging of non-small-cell lung cancer with 18-fluorodeoxyglucose positron-emission tomography. *Thorax* 2001; **56**: (Suppl II): ii38–44.

11. Goldsmith SJ, Kostakoglu L. Role of nuclear medicine in the evaluation of the solitary pulmonary nodule. *Semin Ultrasound CT MRI* 2000; **21**: 129–38.

12. Goldsmith SJ, Kostakoglu L. Nuclear medicine imaging of lung cancer. *Radiol Clin North Am* 2000; **38**: 511–24.

13. McCain TW, Dunagan DP, Chin R Jr et al. The usefulness of positron emission tomography in evaluating patients for pulmonary malignancies. *Chest* 2000; **118**: 1610–15.

14. Dunagan DP, Chin R, McCain TW et al. Staging by positron emission tomography predicts survival in patients with non-small cell lung cancer. *Chest* 2001; **119**: 333–9.

15. Salminen E, MacManus M. FDG–PET imaging in the management of non-small-cell lung cancer. *Ann Oncol* 2002; **13**: 357–60.

16. Fischer BMB, Mortensen J, Højgaard L. Positron emission tomography in the diagnosis and staging of lung cancer: a systematic, quantitative review. *Lancet Oncol* 2001; **2**: 659–66.

17. Imdahl A, Jenkner S, Brink I et al. Validation of FDG positron emission tomography for differentiation of unknown pulmonary lesions. *Eur J Cardio-Thoracic Surg* 2001; **20**: 324–9.

18. Zhuang H, Pourdehnad M, Lambright ES et al. Dual time point 18F-FDG PET imaging for differentiating malignant from inflammatory processes. *J Nucl Med* 2001; **42**: 1412–17.

19. Poncelet AJ, Lonneux M, Coche E et al. PET–FDG scan enhances but does not replace preoperative surgical staging in non-small cell lung carcinoma. *Eur J Cardio-Thorac Surg* 2001; **20**: 468–75.

20. Gupta NC, Tamim WJ, Graeber GG et al. Mediastinal lymph node sampling following positron emission tomography with fluorodeoxyglucose imaging in lung cancer staging. *Chest* 2001; **120**: 521–7.

21. Lee J, Aronchick JM, Alavi A. Accuracy of F-18 fluorodeoxyglucose positron emission tomography for the evaluation of malignancy in patients presenting with new lung abnormalities. *Chest* 2001; **120**: 1791–7.

22. Gupta NC, Graeber GM, Bishop HA. Comparative efficacy of positron emission tomography with fluorodeoxyglucose in evaluation of small (<1 cm), intermediate (1 to 3 cm), and large (>3 cm) lymph node lesions. *Chest* 2000; **117**: 773–8.

23. MacManus MP, Hicks RJ, Matthews JP et al. High rate of detection of unsuspected distant metastases by PET in apparent stage III non-small-cell lung cancer: implications for radical radiation therapy. *Int J Radiat Oncol Biol Phys* 2001; **50**: 287–93.

24. MacManus MP, Hicks RJ, Ball DL et al. F-18 fluorodeoxyglucose positron emission tomography staging in radical radiotherapy candidates with nonsmall cell lung carcinoma. *Cancer* 2001; **92**: 886–95.

25. Mah K, Caldwell CB, Ung YC et al. The impact of 18FDG–PET on target and critical organs in CT-based treatment planning of patients with poorly defined non-small-cell lung carcinoma: a prospective study. *Int J Radiat Oncol Biol Phys* 2002; **52**: 339–50.

26. Akhurst T, Downey RJ, Ginsberg MS et al. An initial experience with FDG–PET in the imaging of residual disease after induction therapy for lung cancer. *Ann Thorac Surg* 2002; **73**: 259–66.

27. Mateu-Navarro M, Rami-Porta R, Bastus-Piulats R et al. Remediastinoscopy after induction chemotherapy in non-small cell

lung cancer. *Ann Thorac Surg* 2000; 70: 391–5.

28. The Canadian Lung Oncology Group. Investigating extrathoracic metastatic disease in patients with apparently operable lung cancer. *Ann Thorac Surg* 2001; 71: 425–34.

29. Mattioli S, D'Ovidio F, Tazzari P et al. Iliac crest biopsy versus rib segment resection for the detection of bone marrow isolated tumor cells from lung and esophageal cancer. *Eur J Cardio-Thorac Surg* 2001; 19: 576–9.

30. Poncelet AJ, Weynand B, Ferdin F et al. Bone marrow micrometastasis might not be a short-term predictor of survival in early stages non-small cell lung carcinoma. *Eur J Cardio-Thorac Surg* 2001; 20: 481–8.

31. Hofmann H-S, Knolle J, Bahn H, Klapperstück T et al. Flow cytometric analysis of DNA content and proliferation and immunohisto-chemical staining of Ki-67 in non-small cell lung cancer. *J Cardiovasc Surg* 2001; 42: 555–60.

32. Steels E, Paesmans M, Berghmans T et al. Role of p53 as a prognostic factor for survival in lung cancer: a systematic review of the literature with a meta-analysis. *Eur Respir J* 2001; 18: 705–19.

33. Kristiansen G, Yu Y, Petersen S et al. Overexpression of *c-erbB2* protein correlates with disease-stage and chromosomal gain at the *c-erbB2* locus in non-small cell lung cancer. *Eur J Cancer* 2001; 37: 1089–95.

34. Gessner C, Liebers U, Kuhn H et al. BAX and p16[INK4A] are independent positive prognostic markers for advanced tumour stage of nonsmall cell lung cancer. *Eur Respir J* 2002; 19: 134–40.

35. González-Quevedo R, Iniesta P, Morán A et al. Cooperative role of telomerase activity and p16 expression in the prognosis of non-small-cell lung cancer. *J Clin Oncol* 2002; 20: 254–62.

36. Arinaga M, Shimizu S, Gotoh K et al. Expression of human telomerase subunit genes in primary lung cancer and its clinical significance. *Ann Thorac Surg* 2000; 70: 401–6.

37. Yuan A, Yu C-J, Kuo S-H et al. Vascular endothelial growth factor 189 mRNA isoform expression specifically correlates with tumor angiogenesis, patient survival, and postoperative relapse in non-small-cell lung cancer. *J Clin Oncol* 2001; 19: 432–41.

38. Müller-Tidow C, Metzger R, Kügler K et al. Cyclin E is the only cyclin-dependent kinase 2-associated cyclin that predicts metastasis and survival in early stage non-small cell lung cancer. *Cancer Res* 2001; 61: 647–53.

39. Salden M, Splinter TW, Peters HA et al. The urokinase-type plasminogen activator system in resected non-small-cell lung cancer. *Ann Oncol* 2000; 11: 327–32.

40. Sasaki H, Auclair D, Fukai I et al. Serum level of the periostin, a homologue of an insect cell adhesion molecule, as a prognostic marker in nonsmall cell lung carcinomas. *Cancer* 2001; 92: 843–8.

41. D'Amico TA, Aloia TA, Moore M-BH et al. Predicting the sites of metastases from lung cancer using molecular biologic markers. *Ann Thorac Surg* 2001; 72: 1144–8.

42. Werle B, Kraft C, Lah TT et al. Cathepsin B in infiltrated lymph nodes is of prognostic significance for patients with nonsmall cell lung carcinoma. *Cancer* 2000; 89: 2282–91.

43. Liu D, Huang C-L, Kameyama K et al. E-cadherin expression associated with differentiation and prognosis in patients with non-small cell lung cancer. *Ann Thorac Surg* 2001; 71: 949–55.

44. Herbst RS, Yano S, Kuniyasu H et al. Differential expression of E-cadherin and type IV collagenase genes predicts outcome in patients

with stage I non-small cell lung carcinoma. *Clin Cancer Res* 2000; **6**: 790–7.

45. Ramnath N, Hernandez FJ, Tan D-F et al. MCM2 is an independent predictor of survival in patients with non-small-cell lung cancer. *J Clin Oncol* 2001; **19**: 4259–66.

46. Saijo Y, Sato G, Usui K et al. Expression of nucleolar protein p120 predicts poor prognosis in patients with stage I lung adenocarcinoma. *Ann Oncol* 2001; **12**: 1121–5.

47. Kakolyris S, Giatromanolaki A, Koukourakis M et al. Thioredoxin expression is associated with lymph node status and prognosis in early operable non-small cell lung cancer. *Clin Cancer Res* 2001; **7**: 3087–91.

48. Hsu N-Y, Ho H-C, Chow K-C et al. Overexpression of dihydrodiol dehydrogenase as a prognostic marker of non-small cell lung cancer. *Cancer Res* 2001; **61**: 2727–31.

49. Tanaka F, Otake Y, Nakagawa T et al. Prognostic significance of polysialic acid expression in resected non-small cell lung cancer. *Cancer Res* 2001; **61**: 1666–70.

50. Ardizzoni A, Cafferata MA, Paganuzzi M et al. Study of pretreatment serum levels of Her-2/*neu* oncoprotein as a prognostic and predictive factor in patients with advanced nonsmall cell lung carcinoma. *Cancer* 2001; **92**: 1896–904.

51. Giatromanolaki A, Koukourakis MI, Sivridis E et al. Relation of hypoxia inducible factor 1α and 2α in operable non-small cell lung cancer to angiogenic/molecular profile of tumours and survival. *Br J Cancer* 2001; **85**: 881–90.

52. Ferrigno D, Buccheri G, Ricca I. Prognostic significance of blood coagulation tests in lung cancer. *Eur Respir J* 2001; **17**: 667–73.

53. Ando M, Ando Y, Hasegawa Y et al. Prognostic value of performance status assessed by patients themselves, nurses, and oncologists in advanced non-small cell lung cancer. *Br J Cancer* 2001; **85**: 1634–9.

54. Montazeri A, Milroy R, Hole D et al. Quality of life in lung cancer patients as an important prognostic factor. *Lung Cancer* 2001; **31**: 233–40.

55. Micke P, Faldum A, Metz T et al. Staging small cell lung cancer: VALG versus IASLC – What limits limited disease? *Lung Cancer* 2002; **37**: 271–6.

56. Hauber HP, Bohuslovizki KH, Lund CH et al. Positron emission tomography in the staging of small-cell lung cancer. *Chest* 2001; **119**: 950–4.

57. Schumacher T, Brink I, Mix M et al. FDG-PET imaging for the staging and follow-up of small cell lung cancer. *Eur J Nucl Med* 2001; **28**: 483–8.

58. Kao A, Shiun SC, Hsu NY et al. Technetium-99m methoxyisobutylisonitrile chest imaging for small-cell lung cancer. *Ann Oncol* 2001; **12**: 1561–6.

59. Giovanella L, Ceriani L, Bandera M, Garancini S. Immunoradiometric assay of chromogranin A in the diagnosis of small cell lung cancer: comparative evaluation with neuron-specific enolase. *Int J Biol Markers* 2001; **16**: 50–5.

60. Castro MP, McDonald TJ, Qualman SJ, Odorisio TM. Cerebrospinal fluid gastrin releasing peptide in the diagnosis of leptomeningeal metastases from small cell carcinoma. *Cancer* 2001; **91**: 2122–6.

61. Tas F, Aydiner A, Demir C, Topuz E. Serum lactate dehydrogenase levels at presentation predict outcome of patients with limited-stage small-cell lung cancer. *Am J Clin Oncol* 2001; **24**: 376–8.

62. Micke P, Hengstler JG, Ros R et al. c-ERBB-2 expression in small-cell lung cancer is associated with poor prognosis. *Int J Cancer* 2001; **92**: 474–9.

6
Treatment of small cell lung cancer

The treatment of small cell lung cancer (SCLC) has been the subject of several reviews, ranging from guidelines developed by the National Comprehensive Cancer Network in the USA,[1] to reviews on the treatment of limited SCLC,[2] to reports on current clinical trials,[3] to a full supplement in *Seminars in Oncology*[4] based on the satellite symposia held in Tokyo, Japan in September 2000 in association with the 9th World Conference on Lung Cancer held by the International Association for the Study of Lung Cancer (IASLC).

The resources used and costs associated with the management of SCLC have also been analyzed in a study from the UK.[5] The main objective of this study was to obtain information on current patterns of care and associated resource use for patients with SCLC from initial diagnosis and treatment phase, throughout disease progression and terminal care. A 4-year retrospective patient chart analysis for the period 1994–1997 was conducted on a consecutive series of 109 patients diagnosed with SCLC in two Newcastle hospitals. The costs were determined from a variety of sources, including the Newcastle Hospitals NHS Trust Finance Department and the British National Formulary. The average total cost per patient calculated for the full cohort of 109 patients was £11 556. Initial treatment was the most resource use-intensive, constituting 48.2% of the total cost. The major cost element throughout all disease phases was hospitalization. Twenty-eight percent of the total costs of care occurred after recurrence of the disease until death, of which 73% were generated by terminal care.

With respect to results on the overall management of SCLC, a study from North America analyzed the trends in survival in patients with limited-stage SCLC from randomized clinical trials performed by cooperative groups in North America initiated between 1972 and 1992 and completed by 1996. Forty-four phase III trials met these criteria; 18 trials were excluded from the analysis because of their small size (<10 patients per arm), because information was lacking on limited-stage SCLC, because prophylactic cranial irradiation was the only study variable, or because randomization was based on response to initial therapy. The median survival in the control arms in 26 phase III studies initiated between 1972 and 1981 was 12 months, and this increased to 17 months between 1982 and 1992 ($p < 0.01$ for trend).[6] Data from the US National Cancer Institute's Surveillance, Epidemiology, and End Results (SEER) database demonstrated a linear 5-month increase in median survival of limited-stage SCLC from 1973 to 1996 ($p \leq 0.001$ for trend). Since 1975, the 5-year survival rate of these patients listed in the SEER database has more than doubled, from 5.2% to 12.2%. The authors concluded that the analysis of these studies and the SEER data show that there has been a significant improvement in the median and 5-year survivals of patients with limited-stage SCLC over the past 20 years. Data from the SEER database have previously indicated that for both stages of SCLC, the median survival has increased by 2 months and the 5-year survival rate by 3.5% ($p \leq 0.001$).

SURGERY

In the very rare case of an SCLC patient presenting with stage I or II disease, surgery is indicated, provided that it is followed by postoperative chemotherapy. Overall, the 5-year survival rate is about 35–40% and patients with no nodal metastases fare better than those who are node-positive. Additional light has been shed on the potential role of surgery by two groups of investigators in Poland. Badzio et al[7] performed a retrospective analysis of survival in two groups of limited-disease SCLC patients treated between 1982 and 1992. One group (67 patients) was managed with complete resection followed by chemotherapy and the other (67 patients) with conventional non-surgical methods. The non-surgical group was selected using a pair-matched case–control method, with 176 patients with limited disease potentially suitable for surgery (e.g. with non-pleural effusion or other local advancement, no supraclavicular lymph node involvement, and good performance status) pre-treated with a non-surgical approach. The total series included 51 N_0, 43 N_1, and 40 N_2 cases. In the surgical group, 23 patients received prophylactic cranial irradiation, and in the non-surgical group, 39 patients received thoracic irradiation. The most important prognostic factors were well balanced between both groups. Median survivals in patients treated with and without surgery were 22 and 11 months, respectively ($p < 0.01$). The 2- and 5-year survival rates were 43% and 27%, respectively, in the surgical group and 17% and 4% in the non-surgical group. Local relapse was more frequent in patients treated conventionally (55%) than in surgically treated patients (15%) ($p < 0.01$). Distant relapses were similar in the two groups: 36% and 40%, respectively. Surgery may thus have a positive impact on the survival of limited-stage SCLC patients, but a randomized study addressing this issue is still needed.

Another Polish study describes a clinical trial that took place between November 1981 and June 1996.[8] Seventy-five patients with stage I–IIIA disease were given etoposide-based cytoreductive chemotherapy. After three courses of induction treatment, 46 patients underwent thoracotomy and 35 of them had resection. Four weeks after surgery, chemotherapy was resumed. Out of 35 patients, 6(17%) had no residual tumor in the resected specimen. Eight patients, mainly with chemotherapy-induced surgicopathologic complete remission and with lymph nodes free of tumor in surgical specimens, are alive, tumor-free, at a median of 136 months or more. There were no long-term survivors among the patients with persistent N_2 disease. The median survival in all 35 patients was 18 months, the 5-year tumor-free survival rate was 29%, and the 10-year tumor-free survival rate was 23%. The results are encouraging, but are based on a highly selected patient material.

Surgery might also be indicated in patients with previously treated SCLC who develop non-small cell lung cancer (NSCLC). Smythe et al[9] analyzed 1404 patients with SCLC at the MD Anderson Hospital in Houston, 29 of whom underwent therapy for metachronous NSCLC: 11 of 29 patients underwent surgical resection; 10 of these 11 were stage I, the majority with squamous cell histology. The SCLC/NSCLC patients had significantly poorer survival when compared with stage I NSCLC patients undergoing any resection (24.5 months versus 74.4 months; $p = 0.003$).

RADIOTHERAPY

Chest irradiation

Radiotherapy of the chest is indicated in cases of limited SCLC because it increases survival and local control. However, a number of issues regarding radiotherapy for this group of patients remain to be solved, such as fractionation, timing, other treatment modalities, dose, and volume of irradiation, as discussed by Curran[10] and also by Tsukada et al,[11] who focused particularly on the issue of concurrent versus sequential radiotherapy. The final decision must obviously consider the patient's pulmonary and cardiac fitness, ability to tolerate specific chemotherapeutic agents, prior history of malignancies and their treatment, as well as patient age and performance status, as pointed out by Curran,[10] who also discuss thoracic radiotherapy dose, altered fractionation radiotherapy, thoracic radiotherapy volume, and chemotherapy selection and dosing in connection with chest irradiation.

With respect to chest irradiation, the Patterns of Care Study (PCS) in Japan conducted a nationwide audit survey in order to establish the national practice process of radiotherapy for SCLC and examined the influence of institutional stratification on the process of care in Japan.[12] The PCS randomly sampled institutions and patients using a two-stage cluster method and surveyed the process of radiotherapy of SCLC patients according to the category of institution. The overall conclusion of this study showed that the use of modern radiotherapy together with chemotherapy mainly took place at academic institutions treating more than 300 patients a year, while this treatment strategy was implemented less often at non-academic institutions seeing less than 120 patients a year.

With respect to the quality of radiotherapy, the North Central Cancer Treatment Group (NCCTG) in the USA[13] has undertaken an analysis of previously published studies applying daily thoracic radiotherapy versus twice-daily thoracic radiotherapy using the Q-TwiST (quality time without symptoms or toxicity). A new graphic representation called a quality-adjusted life-years plot was developed, presenting a complete and concise Q-TwiST analysis on a single plot. The Q-TwiST plot incorporates the time without symptoms or toxicity and several combinations of utility coefficients for toxicity and relapse days into the same plot. In addition, the plot includes threshold lines to judge whether a particular combination of utility coefficients reaches a significance level. This work refines the data previously reported, with the same results – showing no significant difference in survival between daily versus twice-daily administration, after adjusting for toxicity and progression. Because of the discrepancy between the data from the NCCTG and the Eastern Cooperative Oncology Group (ECOG) published by Turrisi et al,[14] the authors suggest that a similar analysis of the recent ECOG trial would be beneficial to determine whether the toxicity of twice-daily thoracic radiotherapy obviates a portion of the survival benefit that was found for this treatment after an appropriate Q-TwiST assessment has been made.

With respect to randomized trials focusing on thoracic irradiation, the literature in 2001 is very scarce. A small randomized study was published by Skarlos et al,[15] who randomized patients with limited SCLC and good performance status to receive hyperfractionated thoracic radiotherapy (HTRT), consisting of 1.5 Gy per fraction daily up to a total dose of 45 Gy, either concurrently with the first cycle (group A) or with the fourth cycle (group B) of chemotherapy. Chemotherapy consisted of carboplatin administered at an area under the curve (AUC) of 6 given as a 1-hour intravenous infusion immediately followed by etoposide at a dose of 100 mg/m^2 as a 2-hour intravenous infusion for 3 consecutive days every 3 weeks up to a total of six cycles. Prophylactic cranial irradiation was also given to patients achieving a complete response. In groups A and B, 42 and 39 patients, respectively, were eligible for efficacy evaluation. The respective overall response rates were 76% and 92.5% in groups A and B, with complete response rates of 40.5% and 56.5%. After a median follow-up of 35 months, the times to progression were 9.5 and 10.5 months in groups A and B, respectively, while the overall median survivals were 17.5 and 17 months. The 2-year survival rates were 36% and 29% in groups A and B, respectively, and the 3-year survival rates were 22% and 13%. The distant relapse rates were 38% and 61% in groups A and B, respectively ($p = 0.046$). Although there was a trend towards a higher response rate in the group of patients who received late HFRT, the overall median, 2-year, and 3-year survival rates did not differ significantly between the two treatment groups. Larger comparative phase III studies with an adequate number of patients are needed in order to answer this question.

The effect of chest irradiation has also been explored in phase II studies using, for example, accelerated hyperfractionated thoracic radiotherapy (AHFTRT) after induction chemotherapy. The radiotherapy consisted of 30 Gy given as 1.5 Gy fractions twice daily with a 2-week break; the AHFTRT was then repeated. The AHFTRT was given concomitantly with daily oral etoposide and cisplatin.[16] The authors claim that the results of their study are similar to those observed with the standard treatment of limited-stage SCLC, but with an interesting low rate of grade III–IV esophagitis (1%) and a low rate of local relapse. However, the treatment-related mortality rate was reported to be 7%.

Other phase II studies have included paclitaxel in combinations with cisplatin and etoposide, together with concurrent radiation or again etoposide and cisplatin, but now combined with ifosfamide.[17,18] The authors of the two studies concluded that the combinations with paclitaxel are effective and well tolerated in patients with limited-stage SCLC,[18] while the ifosfamide regimen failed to demonstrate a superior response rate compared with other series utilizing etoposide and cisplatin; in addition, treatment-related morbidity and mortality appear to be unacceptably high with the ifosfamide regimen.[18] The number of patients allocated to these phase II studies is rather small, prohibiting firm conclusions.

With respect to toxicity, Rosen et al[19] have investigated the relationship between physician-identified radiographic fibrosis, lung tissue physical density change, and radiation dose after concurrent radio- and chemotherapy for limited-stage SCLC. Fibrosis volumes of different severity levels were delineated on computed tomography (CT) images obtained at 1-year follow-up of 21 patients with complete response to concurrent radio- and chemotherapy. The treatments delivered were reconstructed with a three-dimensional (3D) treatment planning system and geometrically registered to the follow-up CT images. Tissue physical density change and radiation dose were computed for each CT image voxel within each fibrosis volume and within normal lung. A significant correlation was noted between fibrosis grade and tissue physical density change and fibrosis grade. For doses of 30–55 Gy and cisplatin and etoposide (PE) chemotherapy, the probability of fibrosis was 2.0 times greater for accelerated fractionation compared with conventional fractionation ($p < 0.005$) and was correlated with increasing dose for both fractionation schedules.

Prophylactic cranial irradiation

Most guidelines recommend the use of prophylactic cranial irradiation (PCI) in limited-stage SCLC patients achieving complete remission based on the meta-analysis published in August 1999 and as discussed in the 2000 *Annual*. In 2001, a Cochrane review study was published re-emphasizing the 1999 meta-analysis.[20] The Cochrane meta-analysis was based on published and unpublished trials and updated individual data. The main endpoint was survival. The results show that the relative risk of death in the treatment group compared with the control group was 0.84 (95% confidence interval, CI, 0.73–0.97; $p = 0.009$), corresponding to a 5.4% increase in the 3-year survival rate from 15.3% in the control group to 20.7% in the treatment group. Prophylactic cranial irradiation also increased disease-free survival (relative risk, RR, 0.75; 95% CI 0.65–0.86; $p < 0.001$) and decreased the risk of brain metastasis (RR

0.46; 95% CI 0.38–0.57; $p < 0.01$). Increasing doses of irradiation decreased the risk of brain metastases when four groups (8, 24–25, 30, and 36–40 Gy) were analyzed (trend test 0.02), but the effect on survival did not differ significantly according to the total dose. The authors found a trend ($p = 0.01$) for a decrease in the brain metastasis risk in favor of early administration of cranial irradiation after the initiation of induction treatment, and concluded that further trials are needed to confirm the potentially greater benefit on brain metastasis rate suggested when cranial irradiation is given earlier or at higher doses. Such studies have now been initiated in Europe with multinational participation, comparing a standard-dose PCI (25 Gy TF/12 days) to a higher dose of conventional radiotherapy (36 Gy in 18 fractions in 24 days) and to accelerated hyperfractionated radiotherapy (36 Gy in 24 fractions in 16 days) in limited-stage SCLC with complete remission. The main endpoint is the brain metastasis rate at 2 years. Quality of life, late sequelae, and survival will also be evaluated. An estimated 700 patients within 3 years will be included in this study, which was activated in September 1999.

Randomized trials on PCI in SCLC have also been reviewed by Kotalik et al[21] from the Cancer Care Ontario Practice Guidelines Initiative Lung Cancer Disease Site Group. Not surprisingly, the results are similar, with the authors again stating that there is insufficient evidence to make a definite recommendation with respect to dose and the optimal timing of PCI in relation to the administration of chemotherapy. There is also insufficient evidence to comment on the long-term effects of PCI on quality of life. The review includes patients in complete remission having either limited or extensive disease, but in the randomized control trials, the majority (> 80%) of patients had limited disease; thus, the data for applying PCI to patients with extensive disease achieving complete remission are still based on insufficient evidence.

PCI has also been subjected to effectiveness and quality of life analyses by Canadian investigators using the Q-TwiST method,[22] similar to the analysis performed for chest irradiation. The analysis again indicates that PCI is a cost-effective treatment that improves the quality-of-life-adjusted survival for patients with complete remission of SCLC.

With respect to schedule, twice-daily PCI has been tested in 15 patients with SCLC in complete remission.[23] The whole brain was treated with twice-daily fractions of 1.5 Gy with megavoltage irradiation to an approximate total dose of 30.0–36.0 Gy. No statistically significant neurologic deterioration was detected in the PCI group post treatment, even though this study was not very detailed. Obviously, a larger phase III trial is needed to evaluate twice-daily PCI in patients with limited-stage SCLC who retain complete remission.

SYSTEMIC TREATMENT

Chemotherapy remains the keystone in the treatment of SCLC, as emphasized in a review article in 2001,[24] when the literature also brought interesting

Table 6.1   Commonest of 23 chemotherapy regimens prescribed for 2262 SCLC patients with good performance status and 49 with limited disease[29]

Regimen	No. of patients
ACE	640 (28%)
IcbE	288 (13%)
CAV	283 (12%)
CbE	277 (12%)
PE	275 (12%)
VAC/PE	197 (9%)
CAVE	183 (8%)
VICbE	36 (2%)
ECMxV	23 (1%)
Other regimens	109 (5%)
Total patients	2311 (100%)

articles on new advances in lung cancer chemotherapy with focus on topotecan, including oral administration of topotecan[25–28] and other topoisomerase I-targeting agents. The most frequently used combination remains etoposide with a platinum compound, often cisplatin. Chemotherapy regimens vary from country to country, and also within the same country, as demonstrated in a study by the UK Medical Research Council Clinical Trials Unit,[29] who conducted a survey among all medical and clinical oncologists, respiratory physicians, and general physicians with respiratory interests in the UK to find out which regimens are used by which specialists and for which type of patient. In this survey, 1214 questionnaires were sent out, and responses were received from 88% of clinicians, 25% of whom treated SCLC with chemotherapy. Of 4674 patients given chemotherapy annually, 36% were given it by clinical oncologists, 30% by medical oncologists, 27% by respiratory physicians, and 7% by general physicians. In all, 34 regimens were reported, with 151 different combinations of dose and schedule. In 2311 good-prognosis patients, 23 regimens were used, the commonest are presented in Table 6.1, while the most common regimens for 1517 poor-prognosis patients are listed in Table 6.2. The main reasons affecting choice of regimen were routine local practice, patients' convenience, quality-of-life considerations, trial results, and cost.

SINGLE-AGENT THERAPY

A summary of new drugs for chemotherapy-naive patients with extensive SCLC has been given by Ettinger,[30] and an overview of single-agent phase II trials in refractory or relapsed patients is given in Table 6.3.[31–36] As noted in the table, the response rate is low, with completely negative results for pegylated liposomal doxorubicin.[31] Taxanes have again shown activity, with

Table 6.2   Commonest of 21 chemotherapy regimens prescribed for 1406 SCLC patients with poor performance status and 111 with extensive disease[29]

Regimen	No. of patients
CAV	544 (36%)
EV	264 (17%)
CbE	137 (9%)
CAV/PE	136 (9%)
Oral E	132 (9%)
CAVE	88 (6%)
ACE	50 (3%)
CE	41 (3%)
Cb	29 (2%)
VIE	25 (2%)
Other regimens	71 (5%)
Total patients	1517 (100%)

response rates of 30% and 36% for paclitaxel[33] and docetaxel,[36] respectively – but in extremely small studies. Similarly, gemcitabine resulted in a partial response in 5 of 36 patients (13%). The activity of ZD0473 is noteworthy; this is a new-generation platinum compound designed to deliver an extended spectrum of antitumor activity and overcome platinum resistance.[35] Two patients were withdrawn because of drug-related adverse events. The compound was given in doses of 120–150 mg/m^2 in 3-week cycles as 1-hour infusions. One complete response was observed and 3 partial responses occurred among a total of 25 patients, of whom 6 were characterized as drug-resistant (relapsed or progressed 8 weeks or sooner following chemotherapy).[35]

A novel approach using a *bcl-2* antisense oligonucleotide G-3919 and paclitaxel was tested by Rudin et al[37] in a pilot study. The dosage of paclitaxel was 150–175 mg/m^2, with G-3139 being administered at a fixed dose of 3 mg/kg daily as an infusion for 7 days every 3 weeks. No objective responses were observed in 12 patients, but 2 had stable disase. A phase II trial is being planned.[37]

Among the new active agents, von Pawel et al[38] performed a comparative study of oral versus intravenous topotecan in patients with chemosensitive SCLC who had relapsed 90 days or more after cessation of initial chemotherapy. The doses were either orally 2.3 mg/m^2/day $\times$ 5 (52 patients) or intravenously 1.5 mg/m^2/day $\times$ 5 (54 patients) every 21 days. The respective response rates were 23% and 15%, and the median survivals 32 and 25 weeks.

COMBINATION CHEMOTHERAPY – PHASE II TRIALS

In 2001, the results of a number of phase II trials including untreated SCLC patients with extensive disease were published, mostly in abstract form

Table 6.3   Single-agent phase II trials in refractory or relapsed SCLC patients

Treatment	No. of patients	No. of responders[a]			Response rate (%)[b]	Comments	Ref
		CR	PR	Total			
Pegylated liposomal doxorubicin (Caelyx) 50 mg/m² i.v. q3wks	14	0	0	0	0 (0–23)	13 of 14 patients responded to first-line therapy	31
Gemcitabine 1000 g/m² on days 1, 8, and 15 of a 4-week schedule	38	0	5	5	13 (6–27)	Median survival 17 weeks	32
Paclitaxel 80 mg/m² i.v. weekly	9	0	4	4	36 (14–79)	Abstract	33
Topotecan 1.5 mg/m² i.v. q3wks	18	0	2	2	11 (1–34)	Abstract, including 4 patients with PS 2–3	34
ZD0473 120–150 mg/m² i.v. q3wks	25	0	4	4	16 (5–36)	Abstract	35
Docetaxel 60–70 mg/m² q3wks	10	1	2	3	30 (7–65)	Abstract	36

[a] CR, complete response; PR, partial response.
[b] 95% confidence interval in parentheses.

(Table 6.4).[39–52] The majority of the trials incorporated new agents together with known active agents, such as etoposide and platinum compounds, as three-drug combinations – some of them with granulocyte colony-stimulating factor (G-CSF) support. In other trials, etoposide was replaced by a new agent or a platinum compound by a new agent. Another approach has been alternating regimens in order to include two active topoisomerase inhibitors (topotecan and etoposide) in the treatment. Combinations of etoposide with topotecan have also been attempted. Response rates of drug combinations are almost all above 50% ranging from 46% to 95% with overlapping 95% confidence intervals for many of the studies, which almost always contain some proportion of patients with complete remissions. With respect to median survival the results from most of the studies range from 7 to 12 months. Intensive developments lie ahead to determine the potential impact of many of these combinations in the overall management of patients with SCLC.

RANDOMIZED TRIALS – CHEMOTHERAPY

The results of a great number of randomized trials on the use of chemotherapy in SCLC were published in 2001, many as full papers, covering various general aspects dealing with both older regimens and combinations with newer cytostatic agents, as well as more specific topics, such as maintenance therapy, intensification, and prevention of toxicity.

Older regimens

An important study was presented at the ECCO meeting in Lisbon in October 2001 by Sundstrøm et al[53] from Norway, who had investigated whether chemotherapy with etoposide and cisplatin (EP) is superior to cyclophosphamide, epirubicin, and vincristine (CEV) in SCLC. In this trial, 436 eligible patients were randomized to chemotherapy with EP (n = 218) or CEV (n = 218). The patients were stratified according to extent of disease (214 with limited disease and 222 with extensive disease). The EP group received five courses of intravenous etoposide 100 mg/m^2 and intravenous cisplatin 75 mg/m^2 on day 1, followed by oral etoposide 200 mg/m^2 daily on days 2–4. The CEV group received five courses of epirubicin 50 mg/m^2, cyclophosphamide 1000 mg/m^2, and vincristine 2 mg, all intravenously on day 1. In addition, limited-disease patients received thoracic radiotherapy concurrent with chemotherapy cycle 3, and those achieving complete remission during the treatment period received prophylactic cranial irradiation. The treatment groups were well balanced. For all patients, the 2- and 5-year survival rates in the EP arm (14% and 5%; p = 0.0004) were significantly higher compared with the CEV arm (6% and 2%). Among limited-disease patients, the median survivals were 14.5 and 9.7 months in the EP and CEV arms respectively (p = 0.001). The 2- and 5-year survival rates were 25% and 10%, respectively,

Table 6.4   Combination chemotherapy in untreated SCLC patients: phase II trials

Treatment	No. of patients	No. of responders[a]			Response rate (%)[b]	Median survival (months)	Survival rate (%)		Comments	Ref
		CR	PR	Total			1-yr	2-yr		
Gemcitabine + etoposide	37	0	17	17	46 (29–63)	10.5	–	–	Median duration of response 5.8 months	39
Topotecan + etoposide	19	4	14	18	95 (74–100)	10.0	–	–	–	40
Paclitaxel + carboplatin	46	3	27	30	65 (51–80)	9	22.5	–	–	41
Paclitaxel + carboplatin	48	3	23	26	54 (39–68)	9.6	–	–	–	42
Cisplatin + paclitaxel + topotecan, + G-CSF support	37	8	22	30	81 (65–92)	12.5	55	21	All patients had extensive disease	43
Cisplatin + paclitaxel + etoposide, + G-CSF support	84	10	38	48	56 (46–68)	11	43	8	–	44
Topotecan + paclitaxel + G-CSF support	14	5	5	10	70 (13–65)	–	–	–	–	45
Paclitaxel + irinotecan + carboplatin	19	8	9	17	89 (67–99)	–	–	–	Abstract	46
Cisplatin + etoposide alternating with topotecan	28	2	17	19	68 (44–81)	–	–	–	Abstract. Median duration of response 5.5 months	47

Table 6.4   Continued

Treatment	No. of patients	No. of responders[a]			Response rate (%)[b]	Median survival (months)	Survival rate (%)		Comments	Ref
		CR	PR	Total			1-yr	2-yr		
Paclitaxel followed by topotecan + G-CSF support	30	3	16	19	73 (43–80)	–	–	–	Abstract	48
Gemcitabine + cisplatin	80	1	44	45	56 (45–67)	9	28		Abstract	49
Paclitaxel + topotecan	17	0	9	9	53 (28–77)	–	–	–	Abstract. Three different dose levels	50
Docetaxel + cisplatin	29	–	–	–	71 (51–87)	7	20	–	Abstract. All patients had extensive disease	51
Cisplatin + etoposide alternating with topotecan	32	5	15	20	63 (46–79)	–	48		Abstract	52

[a] CR, complete response; PR, partial response.
[b] 95% confidence interval in parentheses.

in the EP arm, compared with 8% and 3% in the CEV arm ($p = 0.0001$). For extensive-disease patients, there was no significant survival difference between the treatment arms. The study is a national study covering the majority of patients with SCLC diagnosed in Norway, and thus more representative than many other studies.

Using older drugs, Hirsch et al[54] performed a prospective trial to determine if intensification of the platinum dose by giving cisplatin and carboplatin in combination to patients with SCLC yields higher response rates and survival than carboplatin alone in a rather complicated combination chemotherapy regimen, which is shown in Table 6.5. With respect to the platinum compounds, the doses in arm A were carboplatin (AUC = 4, day 1) plus cisplatin (35 mg/m^2 days 2 and 3), while arm B omitted cisplatin. The other compounds in the combination consisted of teniposide, vincristine, cyclophosphamide, and epirubicin. There were no significant differences in the overall treatment outcome for arm A versus arm B in terms of response rates (72% in both arms), complete response rates (40% and 34%, respectively), or median survival (314 and 294 days, respectively). However, for patients with limited disease, both the complete response rate (54% versus 37%; $p < 0.05$), the overall survival (log-rank test, $p < 0.05$), and the 2-year survival rate (11% versus 6%; $p < 0.05$) were higher in the high-dose platinum arm compared with the carboplatin-alone arm.

An editorial commenting on the article by Berghmans et al[55] refers to two systematic reviews of the role of cisplatin and etoposide in the chemotherapy of SCLC by Mascaux et al[56] and Pujol et al,[57] who both conclude that cisplatin should be considered as a first-choice drug in addition to etoposide for the treatment of SCLC. However, the optimal dosage of cisplatin is not clearly determined. They point out that none of the three randomized trials that have assessed the efficacy of high-dose platinum had an appropriate design, because the dosages of other drugs in the high-dose cisplatin regimen were also increased. In the study by Hirsch et al,[54] the authors conclude that further trials with survival as primary endpoint are now needed to confirm the observation that an increase of platinum dosage results in superior survival (at least in limited disease) and that an optimal design should include three arms: a cisplatin regimen, a carboplatin regimen and a cisplatin-plus-carboplatin regimen. Dosages of each drug should be identical in all arms, and an adequate number of patients should be included to give a sufficient power to detect a survival difference (if any).

In 2001, the full paper comparing the two-drug combination consisting of etoposide plus cisplatin with (PCDE) or without (EP) a combination of epirubicin plus cyclophosphamide in the treatment of extensive-stage SCLC was also published.[58] The study was reviewed in last year's *Annual* based on an abstract, and the data from the full paper are now given in Table 6.5. This trial included 226 patients, with assessment of quality of life according to the EORTC Quality-of-Life Questionnaire. The final publication reemphasizes the superiority of the four-drug combination based on complete and partial

Table 6.5   Randomized trials of chemotherapy in advanced SCLC

Treatment	No. of patients	No. of responders[a]			Response rate (%)[b]	Median survival (months)	Survival rate (%)			Comments[c]	Ref
		CR	PR	Total			1-yr	2-yr	5-yr		
Cisplatin 75 mg/m² day 1, etoposide 100 mg/m² day 1 and 200 mg/m² p.o. days 2–4 q3wks × 5 versus	218	–	–	–	–	LD 14.5	–	14	6 (5-yr)	Abstract, LD patients also received chest irradiation and if complete remission also prophylactic cranial irradiation	53
cyclophosphamide 1000 mg/m² i.v., epirubicin 50 mg/m² i.v., and vincristine 2.6 mg/m² i.v. q3wks × 5	218	–	–	–	–	LD 9.7	–	5	2 (5-yr)		
Carboplatin (AUC = 4) day 1, cisplatin 35 mg/m² days 2+3, teniposide 50 mg/m² days 1–5 vincristine 1.3 mg/m² day 1 q4wks plus cyclophosphamide 3 g/m² day 4 epirubicin 150 mg/m² day 1 + cisplatin, carboplatin, teniposide, vincristine as initial treatment versus	136	55	43	98	72	10	4	–	–	Includes both LD and ED	54
Same treatment without cisplatin	134	45	51	96	72	10	4	–	–	For LD, median survival was 417 versus 327 days (p = 0.039)	

Table 6.5 Continued

Treatment	No. of patients	No. of responders[a]			Response rate (%)[b]	Median survival (months)	Survival rate (%)			Comments[c]	Ref
		CR	PR	Total			1-yr	2-yr	3-yr		
Etoposide 100 mg/m² days 1–3 q4wks, cisplatin 100 mg/m² q4wks	109	14	52	66	68 (p = 0.02)	9.3 (p = 0.0067)	29	–	–	All patients had extensive disease	58
versus											
As above, plus cyclophosphamide 400 mg/m² days 1–3 q4wks, epirubicin 40 mg/m² day 1 q4wks	117	25	64	89	76	10.5	40	–	–		
Cisplatin 60 mg/m² day 1 q4wks, irinotecan 60 mg/m² days 1, 8, 15 q4wks	77	2	63	65	84 (74–92)	12.8	58	19 (p = 0.002)	–	Enrollment terminated early because of superior effect of cisplatin plus irinotecan	60
versus											
Cisplatin 80 mg/m² day 1 q4wks, etoposide 100 mg/m² days 1, 2, 3 q4wks	77	7	45	52	67 (60–78)	11.7	47	11	–		
Paclitaxel 175 mg/m² i.v. day 1, cisplatin 80 mg/m² i.v. day 2, etoposide 80 mg/m² i.v. days 2–4 + G-CSF q4wks	62	2	29	31	50 (37–62)	9.5	38	–	–	Includes both LD and ED. Trial stopped prematurely owing to toxicity	61

Table 6.5   Continued

Treatment	No. of patients	No. of responders[a]			Response rate (%)[b]	Median survival (months)	Survival rate (%)			Comments[c]	Ref
		CR	PR	Total			1-yr	2-yr	3-yr		
versus Cisplatin 80 mg/m² i.v. day 1, etoposide 120 mg/m² i.v. days 1–3 q4wks	71	3	31	34	48 (36–50)	10.5	37	–	–		
Paclitaxel 175 mg/m² i.v. day 4, etoposide phosphate 125 mg/m² i.v. days 1–3 q3wks, carboplatin AUC 5 i.v. day 4	306	–	–	–	81.8 (CR 19.3)	–	–	–	–	Abstract. No survival data	62
versus Vincristine 2 mg i.v. days 1, 8, etoposide phosphate 159 mg/m² days 1–3 q3wks, carboplatin AUC 5 + i.v. day 1	309	–	–	–	76.3 (CR 16.6)	–	–	–	–		
Cyclophosphamide 750 mg/m², epirubicin 90 mg/m² q3wks, vincristine 2.0 mg total	25	1	8	9	36 (18–57) ($p > 0.004$)	7	–	–	–	Study still ongoing	63
versus Same as above + low-molecular-weight heparin	25	5	13	18	75 (51–88)	10	–	–	–		

[a] CR, complete response; PR, partial response.
[b] 95% confidence interval in parentheses.
[c] LD, limited disease; ED, extensive disease.

response rates, with those in the PCDE arm being 21% and 55%, respectively, versus 13% and 48% in the EP arm ($p = 0.02$). Patients in the four-drug arm survived longer than those in the two-drug arm (1-year survival rates 40% and 29%, respectively; median survivals 10.5 and 9.3 months, respectively; log-rank $p = 0.0067$). In the Cox model, the relative risk of death for patients in the PCDE arm compared with those in the EP arm was 0.70 (85% confidence interval 0.51–0.95). The disease also progressed more slowly in the PCDE arm. Hematologic toxicity was higher in the PCDE arm, and the toxicity-related death rate was 9% in the four-drug arm versus 5.5% in the EP arm. The publication was accompanied by an editorial entitled: 'Is more better?' by Bruce E Johnson,[59] who is of the opinion that the four-drug regimen should not be adopted as the new standard treatment at present. Johnson's concern is that a 3-week schedule of cisplatin and etoposide rather than 4-week schedule might result in a similar survival. He also points out that the inclusion of hematopoietic colony-stimulating factors with the four-drug regimen could reduce the hospitalization rate for febrile neutropenia and fatal toxicity to make the regimen more tolerable. This modification would likely show up as an improved quality of life or prolongation of survival.

Newer regimens

Among the phase III trials incorporating the new agents, the study by the Japan Clinical Oncology Group[60] discussed in last year's *Annual* comparing cisplatin plus irinotecan versus cisplatin and etoposide has now been published in a peer-reviewed journal. The enrolment into the study was stopped in accordance with the recommendations by the monitoring committee based on the second interim analysis because a statistically significant difference was found in survival. The final data shows a 2-year survival rate of 58% versus 47% and a 3-year survival rate of 19% versus 11% in favor of the cisplatin–irinotecan regimen versus the cisplatin–etoposide regimen.

Among the other new agents, paclitaxel has been evaluated in two randomized trials. In the first, by the Greek Lung Cancer Cooperative Group,[61] 133 chemotherapy-naive patients with limited or extensive stage SCLC were randomized to receive either paclitaxel 175 mg/m^2 by 3-hour intravenous infusion on day 1 and cisplatin 80 mg/m^2 intravenously on day 2 and etoposide 80 mg/m^2 intravenously on days 2–4, with G-CSF support (µg/kg subcutaneously on days 5–15) or cisplatin 80 mg/m^2 intravenously on day 1 and etoposide 120 mg/m^2 intravenously on days 1–3 in cycles every 28 days. Owing to excessive toxicity and mortality observed in the paclitaxel arm, an early interim analysis was performed and the study was closed. Overall, both regimens were equally active based on complete and partial response rates, 1-year survival, and overall survival. There were eight toxic deaths in the paclitaxel arm versus none in the EP arm ($p = 0.001$). In addition, the paclitaxel regimen was associated with more severe toxicity than the etoposide regimen in terms of grade 4 neutropenia, grade 3–4 thrombocytopenia, diarrhea, asthenia, and neurotoxicity.

In the other paclitaxel trial,[62] paclitaxel was combined with etoposide phosphate and carboplatin and compared with a combination of carboplatin, etoposide phosphate, and vincristine instead of paclitaxel. The doses of the various agents are listed in Table 6.5. Altogether, 650 chemonaive patients were included, and both groups were well balanced, with 50% stage I–IIIB patients and 50% stage IV patients in each group. There were no statistically significant differences between the two groups on comparing response rates, which were 81.8% (complete response rate, CR, 19.3%) in group A and 76.3% (CR 16.6%) in group B. No survival data are yet available from the study, which has been presented only in abstract form.

Finally, a study exploring the effect of low-molecular-weight heparin combined with combination chemotherapy has been reported in abstract form, and the trial is still ongoing.[63]

Maintenance therapy

Two studies tested the efficacy of maintenance therapy in patients with extensive-stage SCLC, both trials using topoisomerase inhibitors (Table 6.6). Hanna et al[64] performed a phase III study to determine whether the addition of 3 months of oral etoposide in non-progressing patients with extensive SCLC treated with four cycles of etoposide plus ifosfamide plus cisplatin (VIP) improves progression-free survival or overall survival. All patients received etoposide 75 mg/m^2, ifosfamide 1.2 g/m^2, and cisplatin 20 mg/m^2 intravenously on days 1–4 every 3 weeks for four cycles. Non-progressing patients were randomized to oral etoposide 50 mg/m^2 for 21 consecutive days every 4 weeks for three courses versus no further therapy until progression. From 1993 to 1998, 233 patients were entered and treated with VIP, with 144 non-progressing patients subsequently randomized to oral etoposide ($n = 72$) or observation ($n = 72$). The minimum follow-up for all patients is 2 years. Toxicity with oral etoposide was mild. There was an improvement in median progressive-free survival favoring the maintenance arm of 8.23 months versus 6.5 months ($p = 0.0018$). There was a trend towards an improvement in median survival (12.2 months versus 11.2 months) and in 1-, 2-, and 3-year survival rates (51.4% versus 40.3%, 16.7% versus 6.9%, and 9.1% versus 1.9%, respectively) ($p = 0.0704$) favoring the maintenance arm. The trend was thus clearly in favor of the maintenance arm.

In the other trial,[65] patients with extensive SCLC received four cycles of cisplatin and etoposide, and patients who had not progressed were eligible to be randomized to either observation or further therapy with topotecan. The dose of cisplatin was 60 mg/m^2 over 30 minutes to 2 hours on day 1 and that of etoposide 120 mg/m^2 on days 1, 2, and 3 of a 21-day cycle. The maintenance dose of topotecan was 1.5 mg/m^2 intravenously for 5 days every 21 days. A total of 402 patients were registered, and 223 patients were eligible for randomization to observation or four cycles of topotecan (observation $n = 111$; topotecan $n = 112$). The median survival for all 402 eligible patients

Table 6.6 Maintenance therapy in SCLC: randomized trials

Treatment	No. of patients	No. of responders[a]			Response rate (%)	Median survival (months)	Survival rate (%)			Comments	Ref
		CR	PR	Total			1-yr	2-yr	3-yr		
Cisplatin 20 mg/m² i.v. days 1–4 + ifosfamide 1.2 g/m² i.v. × 4 + etoposide 75 mg/m² i.v. • Etoposide 50 mg/m² daily in 21 days q4wks × 3	72	–	–	–	–	12.2	51.4	16.7	9.1	Progression-free survival from day of treatment 8.2 months versus 6.5 months ($p = 0.0018$)	64
• Observation	72	–	–	–	–	11.2	40.3	6.9	1.9		
Cisplatin 60 mg/m² day 1 × 4 q3wks + etoposide 120 mg/m² i.v. days 1–3 • Topotecan 1.5 mg/m² i.v. q3wks × 4	112	2	6	8	7		28			Progression-free survival from date of randomization 3.6 months versus 2.3 months ($p \le 0.001$)	65
• Observation	111	–	–	–	–		25				

[a] CR, complete response; PR, partial response.

was 9.6 months. The progression-free survival from the date of randomization was significantly better with topotecan compared with observation (3.6 months versus 2.3 months; $p < 0.001$). However, the overall survival from date of randomization was not significantly different between the arms (8.9 months versus 9.3 months; $p = 0.43$). No difference in quality of life between topotecan and observation was observed. The maintenance thus improved progression-free survival but failed to improve overall survival or quality of life.

Intensity of treatment

A follow-up of a previously reported study involving 105 patients with limited-stage SCLC using higher initial doses of cyclophosphamide and cisplatin has been reported.[66] The study was stopped early on the recommendation of an independent data-monitoring committee, and the median duration of follow-up at the time of publication was 33 months. An evaluation after a median follow-up period of 11 years has now taken place, and the recent follow-up results are consistent with previously published findings demonstrating that moderate increases in the initial doses of drugs may lead to a significant improvement in long-term survival among patients with limited SCLC (Figure 6.1).[66]

Intensification of drug doses with accelerated chemotherapy has been tested in patients with limited and extensive disease. Woll et al[67] randomized SCLC patients with a favorable prognosis to either six cycles of ifosfamide, carboplatin, and etoposide (ICE) at 4-week (standard treatment) or 2-week (intensified treatment) intervals. Intensified treatment was supported by daily subcutaneous G-CSF (filgrastim) injections and reinfusion of 750 ml of autologous blood collected immediately before each cycle. Fifty consecutive patients were randomized to standard ($n = 25$) or intensified ($n = 25$) ICE. A total of 94% completed at least three treatment cycles, and 70% completed six cycles; 96% of treatments were given at full dose. The planned dose intensity was 1.0 for standard and 2.0 for intensified ICE. Febrile neutropenia was more common on the standard arm (84% versus 56%), resulting in more days of intravenous antibiotics. Sequential reinfusion of hematopoietic progenitors in whole blood can safely support substantial increases in dose intensity. However, the treatment results were disappointing, with no statistically significant difference between the treatment arms in time to disease progression (272 days for standard versus 327 days for intensified) or in overall survival (355 days versus 371 days).

The European Lung Cancer Working Party have published their results of a three-arm phase III randomized trial, again using accelerated chemotherapy.[68] Patients with extensive-stage SCLC were randomized between the three following arms: (A) standard chemotherapy with six courses of EVI (epirubicin 60 mg/m^2, vindesine 3 mg/m^2, and ifosfamide 5 g/m^2); all drugs

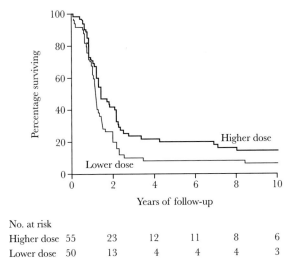

Figure 6.1

Overall survival among patients with limited-stage SCLC according to treatment (higher versus lower initial doses of chemotherapy). From Arriagada R, Pignon J-P, Le Chevalier T. Initial chemotherapeutic doses and long-term survival in limited small-cell lung cancer. *N Engl J Med* 2001; **345:** 1281–2. © 2001 Massachussetts Medical Society. All rights reserved.

being given on day 1 and repeated every 3 weeks; (B) accelerated chemotherapy with EVI administered every 2 weeks and granulocyte–macrophage colony-stimulating factor (GM-CSF) support; (C) accelerated chemotherapy with EVI and oral antibiotics (trimethoprim–sulfamethoxazole (co-trimoxazole)). This trial randomized 233 eligible patients. Chemotherapy could be significantly accelerated in arm B with increased absolute dose intensity. The response rate was significantly higher in arm B compared with arm A; however, again there was no survival difference with respect to median duration and 2-year survival rate of 286 days and 5% for arm A, 264 days and 6% for arm B, and 264 days and 6% for arm C. The trial thus failed to demonstrate in extensive-stage SCLC a survival benefit of chemotherapy acceleration using GM-CSF support.

Prevention of toxicity

In order to prevent chemotherapy-induced febrile leukopenia, the European Organization for Research and Treatment of Cancer (EORTC) Lung Cancer

Group evaluated the impact of prophylactic antibiotics during chemotherapy for SCLC.[69] Patients with SCLC were randomized to standard-dose CDE chemotherapy (cyclophosphamide 1000 mg/m^2 on day 1, doxorubicin 45 mg/m^2 on day 1, intravenous etoposide 100 mg/m^2 on days 1–3, every 3 weeks × 5) or to intensified CDE chemotherapy (125% dose every 2 weeks, × 4, with G-CSF (filgrastim) 5 μg/kg/day on days 4–13) to assess the impact on survival. Patients were also randomized to prophylactic antibiotics (ciprofloxacin 750 mg plus roxithromycin 150 mg, twice daily on days 4–13) or to placebo in a 2 × 2 factorial design (the first 163 patients). Prophylactic ciprofloxacin plus roxithromycin during CDE chemotherapy reduced the incidence of febrile leukopenia, the number of infections, the use of therapeutic antibiotics, and hospitalizations due to febrile leukopenia by approximately 50%, with a reduced number of infectious deaths. The authors concluded that with similar risks for febrile leukopenia, the prophylactic use of antibiotics should be considered.

In a commentary by Bunn,[70] the view is that the data do not justify the prophylactic use of these antibiotics in any SCLC patients. The results of the randomization to standard or intensified CDE chemotherapy are not known, and this conclusion could change if there is benefit for the intensified regimen. Bunn points out that the intensified therapy with G-CSF and prophylactic antibiotics is costly and toxic, and should not be used outside a clinical trial setting – but, as mentioned, this could change if there is a large survival advantage for the intensified arm.

Another randomized trial was conducted to determine whether administration of amifostine with chemotherapy for SCLC could decrease toxicity.[71] In this trial, 84 patients with favorable-prognosis SCLC received treatment with intravenous ifosfamide 3 g/m^2, intravenous carboplatin (glomerular filtration rate + 25) × 6 mg, and oral etoposide 50 mg twice daily for 7 days every 3 weeks. Patients were randomized to receive amifostine 740 mg/m^2 immediately prior to the intravenous drugs (n = 42) or to receive chemotherapy alone (n = 42). The two groups were similar with respect to baseline prognostic factors. There was no significant difference in the occurrence of grade 3 or 4 neutropenia or thrombocytopenia between the two groups, nor in the response rate or overall survival, for which the median was 11 months in the chemotherapy-only group and 14 months in the group treated with amifostine. The study did not show a protective effect from the use of amifostine with this regimen, and there does not appear to be any effect upon the efficacy of treatment.

SPECIAL TOPICS

Relapsed SCLC

More than 90% with SCLC relapse after initial treatment and the overall expected survival post relapse is rather short. No standard treatment or guide-

Table 6.7   Combination chemotherapy in previously treated SCLC patients: phase II trials

Treatment	No. of patients	No. of responders[a]			Response rate (%)[b]	Comments	Ref
		CR	PR	Total			
Paclitaxel + ifosfamide + cisplatin	33	8	16	24	73 (55–87)	1-yr survival rate 12%	72
Paclitaxel + carboplatin	32	1	7	22	25 (10–40)	All patients had extensive disease	73
Paclitaxel + gemcitabine	20	0	10	10	50 (27–73)	Abstract. Median of duration response 5 months	74
Lomustine + cyclophosphamide + etoposide	13	4	3	7	54 (25–81)	Abstract. Orally administered 2nd- and 3rd-line treatment	75

[a] CR, complete response; PR, partial response.
[b] 95% confidence interval in parentheses.

lines exist, and combination chemotherapy has been the standard unless local relapse dominates. In the latter case, radiotherapy is indicated, provided that it has not been applied before.

In contrast to last year, no randomized trials have been published dealing with the treatment of relapsed SCLC, but the literature includes four phase II trials (Table 6.7). Three of the trials include paclitaxel combined with ifosfamide plus cisplatin or carboplatin or gemcitabine. The response rate varied from 25% to 73%, with overlapping 95% confidence intervals. The median duration of response ranged from 5 to 8 months. The more definitive role of these combinations awaits comparative randomized trials, including impact on quality of life. An interesting abstract has been published by Lebeau et al,[75] who used oral drugs: lomustine (CCNU), cyclophosphamide, and etoposide. Surprisingly, four of seven patients achieved a complete remission, even when the combination was used as second- and third-line therapy. One awaits with interest the results of an expansion of this study where this combination is compared with cytostatic agents given intravenously.

Treatment of elderly patients

A special group of SCLC patients consists of elderly patients and those who have decreased organ functions and performance at the time of diagnosis. It is estimated that 25% of patients with SCLC are 70 years of age or older and 10–15% of patients present with poor performance status.

The management of SCLC in the elderly has been extensively reviewed by Gridelli et al,[76] who concluded that in the elderly it is usually difficult to administer the same chemotherapy as in younger patients, and that one needs to design specific trials in order to develop an active and well-tolerated chemotherapy regimen for SCLC in elderly patients. With respect to radiotherapy added to chemotherapy, the intensity of radiotherapy must be accurately evaluated considering the slight survival improvement and the potential related toxicity.

Two French groups have tested the combination of carboplatin and etoposide in elderly patients with SCLC. Larive et al,[77] on behalf of the Groupe Lyon–Saint Etienne d'Oncologie Thoracique, gave intravenous carboplatin on day 1 (AUC 5 using Calvert's formula) and oral etoposide 100 mg/m^2 on days 1–5, every 4 weeks, and thoracic irradiation to limited-disease patients after chemotherapy. The overall response rate was 59% (95% confidence interval 43–76%) and the median survival for all patients was 37 weeks (range 3–76 weeks). The toxicity was mainly hematologic, with grade 3–4 neutropenia in 59% of courses, febrile neutropenia in 15% of courses, and toxic death in 9% of patients. The results of this regimen were disappointing with more hematologic toxicity than expected and previously reported. Possible explanations could be the use of oral rather than intravenous etoposide, the frequent comorbidities of older patients, and the inclusion of patients with poor prognostic factors.

Quoix et al[78] also used a combination of carboplatin for a target AUC value of 5 mg/ml/min. Etoposide was given intravenously on days 1, 2, and 3 at a dose of 100 mg/m^2. Cycles of chemotherapy were repeated at 4-week intervals. Chest irradiation was not routinely applied. There were 2 complete and 20 partial responses in 38 patients evaluated for efficacy, and the median survival was 237 days and the 1-year survival rate 26%. Quoix et al concluded that the combination is feasible in most elderly patients, with acceptable toxicity, and the overall results suggest that patients even older than 70 years may benefit from full treatment. As stressed by Gridelli et al,[76] specific randomized trials are needed in this group of patients – as also emphasized in a commentary by Murray,[79] who pointed out that clinically relevant measures of comorbidity need to be developed and incorporated into these clinical trials. More than age alone, a better accounting of comorbidity in the data should allow us to balance probabilities of benefit and toxicity.

In patients with poor prognostic factors, White et al[80] compared a drug combination using cyclophosphamide, doxorubicin, and vincristine (CAV) versus single-agent carboplatin given at an AUC of 7. The dose in the CAV regimen was intravenous cyclophosphamide 750 mg/m^2, intravenous vincristine 1.3 mg/m^2 (to a maximum of 2 mg), and doxorubicin 40 mg/m^2, all given as a bolus on day 1. Carboplatin was given at 4-week intervals. Patients who had limited disease and an objective response to treatment were considered for consolidation thoracic and prophylactic cranial irradiation. CAV was given to 59 patients, while 60 received carboplatin. As expected, grade 3–4 neutropenia and intravenous antibiotic use were significantly more common with the CAV regimen, while conversely grade 3–4 thrombocytopenia was more common ($p = 0.0009$) and platelet transfusion was more frequent ($p < 0.05$) with carboplatin therapy. Non-hematologic toxicity was similar in both treatment arms. Patients had a Karnofsky score ≤ 50 and/or a prognostic score indicative of a 1-year survival rate below 15%. Symptom relief occurred in 48% and 41% in the CAV and carboplatin arms, respectively. CAV therapy produced a higher response rate than carboplatin (38% versus 25%), but this was not statistically significant ($p = 0.15$). The median overall survivals for patients in the CAV and carboplatin treatment arms were 17 weeks and 15.9 weeks, respectively, with 1-year survival rates of 12% and 6%.

Other neuroendocrine tumors

The spectrum of neuroendocrine neoplasms of the lung has been reviewed by Cooper et al,[81] with emphasis on histopathologic classification and surgical therapy of each class of neoplasms. A total of 77 patients in a 10-year period underwent lung resections, including the following neuroendocrine neoplasms: typical carcinoids (TC) 50 patients, atypical carcinoids (AC) 5 patients, large cell neuroendocrine carcinomas (LCNEC) 9 patients, mixed large/small neuroendocrine carcinomas (LSNEC) 4 patients, and small neuroendocrine carcinomas (SCC) 9 patients. There were 48% men and 51.9% females, with a median age of 57.9 years (range 14–78 years). The hospital mortality rate was 2.6% (2 of 77 patients), and both patients died of pulmonary failure. Follow-up was obtained in 62 (77%) of patients, for an average of 38.1 months (range 2–132 months). There were 13 deaths in all, 8 of which were disease-related (LCNEC 4 deaths, SCC 2 deaths, LSNEC 1 death, and AC 1 death. The mean disease-free intervals for patients with these neoplasms were as follows: TC 41.3 months, AC 22 months, LCNEC 20.4 months, LSNEC 25 months, and SCC 25 months. The overall 3-year survival rate was 45.2% (28 of 62 patients).

Iyoda et al[82] present results with adjuvant chemotherapy using cisplatin, carboplatin, or cyclophosphamide in patients with large cell carcinoma with neuroendocrine features. The number of patients was too small to allow any firm conclusions to be drawn.

The experience in the treatment of metastatic pulmonary carcinoid tumors has been presented by Grandberg et al,[83] based on 31 patients receiving interferon-α or -γ as a single agent or combined with various types of cytostatic agents or various chemotherapy regimens (e.g. cisplatin plus etoposide, or streptozotocin plus 5-fluorouracil or doxorubicin). In addition, some patients have also received paclitaxel. Again, because of the heterogeneity of the treatments, no firm conclusions can be drawn regarding the best choice of systemic antitumor treatment of pulmonary carcinoids with distant metastases.

Other treatments

Alternatives to chemotherapy and radiotherapy for SCLC have been extensively reviewed by Shepherd.[84] These treatments include monoclonal antibody therapy and the use of interferons as adjuvant therapy, but none of the trials showed a significant prolongation of survival. Tumor vaccines against gangliosides, which are expressed on almost all human cells, have also been developed recently. An anti-idiotypic monoclonal antibody against the GD3 ganglioside, BEC-2, is being evaluated after chemotherapy in SCLC patients in a European study. In North America, a bivalent ganglioside vaccine, BMS-248967, is under study at the phase II level. Other new approaches have yet to be shown to have a role to play in the routine management of patients with SCLC.

REFERENCES

1. Johnson BE. Small cell lung cancer. *Cancer Control* 2001; 8(Suppl 2): 32–43.

2. Turisi AT, Sherman CA. The treatment of limited small cell lung cancer: a report of the progress made and future prospects. *Eur J Cancer* 2002; 38: 279–91.

3. Saxman SB, West PJ, Cheson BD. Clinical trials. Referral resource. *Oncology* 2001; 15: 318–23.

4. Greco FA, Saijo N. Introduction. *Semin Oncol* 2001; 28(Suppl 4): 1–2.

5. Oliver E, Killen J, Kiebert G et al. Treatment pathways, resource use and costs in the management of small cell lung cancer. *Thorax* 2001; 56: 785–90.

6. Janne PA, Freidlin B, Saxman S et al. The survival of patients treated for limited stage small cell lung cancer in North America has increased during the past 20 years. *Proc ASCO* 2001; 20: 317a (Abst 1264).

7. Badzio A, Jassem J, Kurowski K, Karnicka-Mlodkowska H. The role of surgery in limited disease (LD) small cell lung cancer (SCLC): a retrospective, comparative study. *Proc ECCO* 2001; 37(Suppl 6): S61 (Abst 216).

8. Lewinski T, Zulawski M, Turski C, Pietraszek A. Small cell lung cancer I–III A: cytoreductive chemotherapy followed by resection with continuation of chemotherapy. *Eur J Cardio-Thorac Surg* 2001; 20: 391–8.

9. Smythe WR, Estrera AL, Swisher SG et al. Surgical resection of non-small cell carcinoma after treatment for small cell carcinoma. *Ann Thorac Surg* 2001; 71: 962–6.

10. Curran WJ. Combined-modality therapy for limited-stage small cell lung cancer. *Semin Oncol* 2001; 28(Suppl 4): 14–22.

11. Tsukada H, Yokoyama A, Goto K et al. Concurrent versus sequential radiotherapy for small cell lung cancer. *Semin Oncol* 2001; 28(Suppl 4): 23–6.

12. Uno T, Sumi M, Ikeda H et al. Radiation therapy for small cell lung cancer: results of the 1995–1997 patterns of care process survey in Japan. *Lung Cancer* 2002; 35: 279–85.

13. Sloan JA, Bonner JA, Hillman SL et al. A quality-adjusted reanalysis of a phase III trial comparing once-daily thoracic radiation vs. twice-daily thoracic radiotherapy in patients with limited-stage small-

cell lung cancer. *Int J Radiat Oncol Biol Phys* 2002; **52**: 371–82.

14. Turrisi AT, Kim K, Blum R et al. Twice daily compared with once daily radiotherapy in limited small cell lung cancer treated concurrently with cisplatin and etoposide. *N Engl J Med* 1999; **340**: 265–71.

15. Skarlos DV, Samantas E, Briassoulis E et al. Randomized comparison of early versus late hyperfractionated thoracic irradiation concurrently with chemotherapy in limited disease small-cell lung cancer: A randomized phase II study of the Hellenic Cooperative Oncology Group (HeCOG). *Ann Oncol* 2001; **12**: 1231–8.

16. Brown PD, Bonner JA, Foote RL et al. Long-term results of a phase I/II study of high-dose thoracic radiotherapy with concomitant cisplatin and etoposide in limited stage small-cell lung cancer. *Am J Clin Oncol* 2001; **24**: 556–61.

17. Bremnes RM, Sundstrøm S, Vilsvik J et al. Multicenter phase II trial of paclitaxel, cisplatin, and etoposide with concurrent radiation for limited-stage small cell lung cancer. *J Clin Oncol* 2001; **19**: 3532–8.

18. Hanna N, Ansari R, Fisher W et al. Etoposide, ifosfamide and cisplatin (VIP) plus concurrent radiation therapy for previously untreated limited small cell lung cancer (SCLC): a Hoosier Oncology Group (HOG) phase II study. *Lung Cancer* 2002; **35**: 293–7.

19. Rosen II, Fischer TA, Antolak JA et al. Correlation between lung fibrosis and radiation therapy dose after concurrent radiation therapy and chemotherapy for limited small cell lung cancer. *Radiology* 2001; **221**: 614–22.

20. The Prophylactic Cranial Irradiation Overview Collaborative Group. Cranial irradiation for preventing brain metastases of small cell lung cancer in patients in complete remission (Cochrane Review).

In: *The Cochrane Library*, Issue 1. Oxford: Update Software, 2001.

21. Kotalik J, Yu E, Markman BR et al. Practice guideline on prophylactic cranial irradiation in small-cell lung cancer. *Int J Radiat Oncol Biol Phys* 2001; **50**: 309–16.

22. Tai THP, Yu E, Dickof P et al. Prophylactic cranial irradiation revisited: cost-effectiveness and quality of life in small-cell lung cancer. *Int J Radiat Oncol Biol Phys* 2002; **52**: 68–74.

23. Wolfson AH, Bains Y, Lu J et al. Twice-daily prophylactic cranial irradiation for patients with limited disase small-cell lung cancer with complete response to chemotherapy and consolidative radiotherapy. *Am J Clin Oncol* 2001; **24**: 290–5.

24. Østerlind K. Chemotherapy in small cell lung cancer. *Eur Respir J* 2001; **18**: 1026–43.

25. Huang CH, Treat J. New advances in lung cancer chemotherapy: topotecan and the role of topoisomerase I inhibitors. *Oncology* 2001; **61**(Suppl 1): 14–24.

26. Ohe Y, Saijo N. Topoisomerase I targeting agents in small-cell lung cancer. *Curr Oncol Rep* 2001; **3**: 170–8.

27. Schiller JH. Future role of topotecan in the treatment of lung cancer. *Oncology* 2001; **61**(Suppl 1): 55–9.

28. Eckardt JR. Feasibility of oral topotecan in previously untreated patients with small-cell lung cancer ineligible for standard therapy. *Oncology* 2001; **61**(Suppl 1): 42–6.

29. Sambrook RJ, Girling DJ. A national survey of the chemotherapy regimens used to treat small cell lung cancer (SCLC) in the United Kingdom. *Br J Cancer* 2001; **84**: 1447–52.

30. Ettinger DS. New drugs for chemotherapy-naïve patients with extensive-disease small cell lung cancer. *Semin Oncol* 2001; **28**: 27–9.

31. Samantas E, Kalofonos H, Linardou H et al. Phase II study of pegylated liposomal doxorubicin: inactive in recurrent small-cell lung cancer. *Ann Oncol* 2000; **11**: 1395–7.

32. van der Lee I, Smit EF, van Putten JWG et al. Single-agent gemcitabine in patients with resistant small-cell lung cancer. *Ann Oncol* 2001; **12**: 557–61.

33. Tukiyama S, Yamamoto N, Uezima H et al. Phase II study of weekly paclitaxel in platinum-treated patients with small cell lung cancer. *Proc ASCO* 2001; **20**: 281b (Abst 2876).

34. Fernandez-Rodriguez R, Ferreiro J, Rubio I et al. Topotecan (TPT) as second-line treatment in small cell lung cancer. *Proc ASCO* 2001; **20**: 283b (Abst 2883).

35. Bonomi P, Modiano M, Cornett P, Koehler M, Schiller J. Phase II trial to assess the activity of ZD0473 in patients with small-cell lung cancer who have failed one prior platinum-based chemotherapy regimen. *Proc ASCO* 2001; **20**: 322a (Abst 1284).

36. Nakamura H, Azuma M, Miyagi K et al. A pilot study of docetaxel (TXT) as salvage chemotherapy in small cell lung cancer (SCLC). *Proc ASCO* 2001; **20**: 280b (Abst 2872).

37. Rudin CM, Otterson GA, Mauer AM et al. A pilot trial of G3139, a *bcl-2* antisense oligonucleotide, and paclitaxel in patients with chemorefractory small-cell lung cancer. *Ann Oncol* 2002; **13**: 539–45.

38. von Pawel J, Gatzemeier U, Pujol J-L et al. Phase II comparator study of oral versus intravenous topotecan in patients with chemosensitive small-cell lung cancer. *J Clin Oncol* 2001; **19**: 1743–9.

39. Vansteenkiste J, Gatzemeier U, Manegold C et al. Gemcitabine plus etoposide in chemonaive extensive disease small-cell lung cancer: a multi-centre phase II study. *Ann Oncol* 2001; **12**: 835–50.

40. O'Neill P, Clark PI, Smith D et al. A phase I trial of a 5-day schedule of intravenous topotecan and etoposide in previously untreated patients with small-cell lung cancer. *Oncology* 2001; **61**(Suppl 1): 25–9.

41. Thomas P, Castelnau O, Paillotin D et al. Phase II trial of paclitaxel and carboplatin in metastatic small-cell lung cancer: a Groupe Francais de Pneumo-Cancérologie study. *J Clin Oncol* 2001; **19**: 1320–5.

42. Gridelli C, Manzione L, Perrone F et al. Carboplatin plus paclitaxel in extensive small cell lung cancer: a multicentre phase 2 study. *Br J Cancer* 2001; **84**: 38–41.

43. Frasci G, Nicolella G, Comella P et al. A weekly regimen of cisplatin, paclitaxel and topotecan with granulocyte-colony stimulating factor support for patients with extensive disease small cell lung cancer: a phase II study. *Br J Cancer* 2001; **84**: 1166–71.

44. Kelly K, Lovato L, Bunn PA Jr. et al. Cisplatin, etoposide, and paclitaxel with granulocyte colony-stimulating factor in untreated patients with extensive-stage small cell lung cancer: a phase II trial of the Southwest Oncology Group. *Clin Cancer Res* 2001; **7**: 2325–9.

45. Schütte W, Bork I, Öhlmann K et al. Phase II study: first line treatment of stage IV small cell lung cancer with topotecan and paclitaxel. *Proc ASCO* 2001; **20**: 283B (Abst 2882).

46. Glisson SD, LaRocca RV, Hargis JB et al. Paclitaxel, irinotecan, and carboplatin (PIC) are effective in treating extensive stage small cell lung cancer: early results of a phase II study. *Proc ASCO* 2001; **20**: 321a (Abst 1281).

47. Vassilis G, Veslemes M, Palamidas P et al. A phase II study alternating

cisplatin-etoposide and topotecan administration in patients with extensive stage small cell lung cancer (SCLC). *Proc ASCO* 2001; **20**: 318a (Abst 1269).

48. Felip E, Font A, Rosell R et al. Sequential dose-dense paclitaxel followed by topotecan in untreated extensive small-cell lung cancer (SCLC): a Spanish Lung Cancer Group phase II study. *Proc ASCO* 2001; **20**: 319a (Abst 1271).

49. Israel VP, Chansky K, Gandara D. Southwest Oncology Group trial (SWOG) S9718: a phase II study of gemcitabine plus cisplatin in patients with extensive small cell lung cancer (E-SCLC). *Proc ASCO* 2001; **20**: 316a (Abst 1262).

50. Schnell FM, Birch R, Sysel IA et al. A phase I trial of combined paclitaxel and topotecan for extensive small cell lung cancer. *Proc ASCO* 2001; **20**: 281b (Abst 2877).

51. Lianes P, Moreno-Nogueira JA, Cardenal F et al. Multicenter phase II clinical trial of doxetaxel (D) in combination with cisplatin (P) in first-line chemotherapy for small-cell lung cancer (SCLC) extensive disease: final results. *Proc ASCO* 2001; **20**: 282b (Abst 2881).

52. Mavroudis D, Pavlakou G, Vesleme M et al. A phase II study of the sequential administration of cis-platin–etoposide and topotecan in patients with extensive stage small cell lung cancer (SCLC). *Proc ASCO* 2001; **20**: 281b (Abst 2885).

53. Sundstrøm S, Bremnes RM, Kaasa S, Aamdal S. Cisplatin and etoposide (EP-regimen) is superior to cyclophosphamide, epirubicin, and vincristine (CEV-regimen) in small cell lung cancer: results from a randomized phase III trial with 5 years follow-up. *Eur J Cancer* 2001; **37**: (Suppl 6): S153 (Abst 556).

54. Hirsch FR, Østerlind K, Jeppesen N et al. Superiority of high-dose platinum (cisplatin and carboplatin)

compared to carboplatin alone in combination chemotherapy for small-cell lung carcinoma: a prospective randomised trial of 280 consecutive patients. *Ann Oncol* 2001; **12**: 647–54.

55. Berghmans T, Paesmans M, Sculier JP. The role of cisplatin in the treatment of small-cell lung cancer? *Ann Oncol* 2001; **12**: 585–6.

56. Mascaux C, Paesmans M, Berghmans T et al. A systematic review of the role of etoposide and cisplatin in the chemotherapy of small-cell lung cancer with methodology assessment and meta-analysis. *Lung Cancer* 2000; **30**: 23–36.

57. Pujol J, Carestia L, Daurés JP. Is there a case for cisplatin in the treatment of small-cell lung cancer? A meta-analysis of randomized trials of a cisplatin-containing regimen vs. a regimen without this alkylating agent. *Br J Cancer* 2001; **83**: 8–15.

58. Pujol J-L, Daurès J-P, Rivière A et al. Etoposide plus cisplatin with or without the combination of 4′-epidoxorubicin plus cyclophosphamide in treatment of extensive small-cell lung cancer: a French Federation of Cancer Institutes multicenter phase III randomized study. *J Natl Cancer Inst* 2001; **93**: 300–8.

59. Johnson BE. Is more better? Chemotherapy for patients with extensive-stage small-cell lung cancer. *J Natl Cancer Inst* 2001; **93**: 254–5.

60. Noda K, Nishiwaki Y, Kawahara M et al. Irinotecan plus cisplatin compared with etoposide plus cisplatin for extensive small-cell lung cancer. *N Engl J Med* 2002; **346**: 85–91.

61. Mavroudis D, Papadakis E, Veslemes M et al. A multicenter randomized clinical trial comparing paclitaxel–cisplatin–etoposide versus cisplatin–etoposide as first-

line treatment in patients with small-cell lung cancer. *Ann Oncol* 2001; **12**: 463–70.

62. Reck M, Von Pawel J, Macha H et al. First-line chemotherapy in SCLC: a phase III study of Taxol, etoposide phosphate and carboplatin (TEC) versus carboplatin, etoposide phosphate and vincristin (CEV). *Eur J Cancer* 2001; 37(Suppl 6): S153 (Abst 557).

63. Altinbas M, Coskun H, Er O et al. Prospective randomized study of epirubicine cyclophosphamide and vincristine combination chemotherapy (CEV) ± low molecular weight heparin (LMWH) in small cell lung cancer (SCLC). *Proc ASCO* 2001; **20**: 321a (Abst 1280).

64. Hanna NH, Sandler AB, Loehrer PJ Sr et al. Maintenance daily oral etoposide versus no further therapy following induction chemotherapy with etoposide plus ifosfamide plus cisplatin in extensive small-cell lung cancer: a Hoosier Oncology Group randomized study. *Ann Oncol* 2002; **13**: 95–102.

65. Schiller JH, Adak S, Cella D et al. Topotecan versus observation after cisplatin plus etoposide in extensive-stage small-cell lung cancer: E7593 – a phase III trial of the Eastern Cooperative Oncology Group. *J Clin Oncol* 2001; **19**: 2114–22.

66. Arriagada R, Pignon J-P, Le Chevalier T. Initial chemotherapeutic doses and long-term survival in limited small-cell lung cancer. *N Engl J Med* 2001; **345**: 1281–2.

67. Woll PJ, Thatcher N, Lomax L et al. Use of hematopoietic progenitors in whole blood to support dose-dense chemotherapy: a randomized phase II trial in small cell lung cancer patients. *J Clin Oncol* 2001; **19**: 712–19.

68. Sculier JP, Paesmans M, Lecomte J et al. A three-arm phase III randomised trial assessing, in patients with extensive-disease small-cell

lung cancer, accelerated chemotherapy with support of haematological growth factor or oral antibiotics. *Br J Cancer* 2001; **85**: 1444–51.

69. Tjan-Heijnen VCG, Postmus PE, Ardizzoni A et al. Reduction of chemotherapy-induced febrile leucopenia by prophylactic use of ciprofloxacin and roxithromycin in small-cell lung cancer patients: an EORTC double-blind placebo-controlled phase III study. *Ann Oncol* 2001; **12**: 1359–68.

70. Bunn PA Jr. Editorial comments on 'Reduction of chemotherapy-induced febrile leucopenia by prophylactic use of ciprofloxacin and roxithromycin in small-cell lung cancer patients: an EORTC double-blind placebo-controlled phase III study'. *Ann Oncol* 2001; **12**: 1339–40.

71. Johnson PWM, Muers MF, Peake MD et al. A randomized trial of amifostine as a cytoprotective agent in patients receiving chemotherapy for small cell lung cancer. *Br J Cancer* 2001; **84**: 19–24.

72. Kosmas C, Tsavaris NB, Malamos NA et al. Phase II study of paclitaxel, ifosfamide, and cisplatin as second-line treatment in relapsed small-cell lung cancer. *J Clin Oncol* 2001; **19**: 119–26.

73. Kakolyris S, Mavroudis D, Tsavaris N et al. Paclitaxel in combination with carboplatin as salvage treatment in refractory small-cell lung cancer (SCLC): a multicenter phase II study. *Ann Oncol* 2001; **12**: 193–7.

74. Domine M, Gonzalez Larriba J, Carcia Gomez R et al. Paclitaxel and gemcitabine for refractory or relapsed small cell lung cancer (SCLC). A multicentric phase II study. *Eur J Cancer* 2001; 37(Suppl 6): S62 (Abst 220).

75. Lebeau B, Giraud F, Baud M. Oral chemotherapy by lomustine–etoposide–cyclophosphamide for current

small cell lung cancer. *Proc ASCO* 2001; **20**: 270b (Abst 2874).

76. Gridelli C, De Vivo R, Monfardini S. Management of small-cell lung cancer in the elderly. *Crit Rev Oncol Hematol* 2002; **41**: 79–88.

77. Larive S, Bombaron P, Riou R et al. Carboplatin–etoposide combination in small cell lung cancer patients older than 70 years: a phase II trial. *Lung Cancer* 2002; **35**: 1–7.

78. Quoix E, Breton JL, Daniel C et al. Etoposide phosphate with carboplatin in the treatment of elderly patients with small-cell lung cancer: a phase II study. *Ann Oncol* 2001; **12**: 957–62.

79. Murray N. Commentary on 'Carboplatin–etoposide association in small cell lung cancer patients older than 70 years: a phase II trial'. *Lung Cancer* 2002; **35**: 9–10.

80. White SC, Lorigan P, Middleton MR et al. Randomized phase II study of cyclophosphamide, doxo-rubicin, and vincristine compared with single-agent carboplatin in patients with poor prognosis small cell lung carcinoma. *Cancer* 2001; **92**: 601–8.

81. Cooper WA, Thourani VH, Gal AA et al. The surgical spectrum of pulmonary neuroendocrine neoplasms. *Chest* 2001; **119**: 14–18.

82. Iyoda A, Hiroshima K, Toyozaki T et al. Adjuvant chemotherapy for large cell carcinoma with neuroendocrine features. *Cancer* 2001; **92**: 1108–12.

83. Granberg D, Eriksson B, Wilander E et al. Experience in treatment of metastatic pulmonary carcinoid tumors. *Ann Oncol* 2001; **12**: 1283–91.

84. Shepherd FA. Alternatives to chemotherapy and radiotherapy in the treatment of small cell lung cancer. *Semin Oncol* 2001; **28**(Suppl 4): 30–7.

7

Treatment of non-small cell lung cancer

STAGE I, II, AND RESECTABLE IIIA NSCLC

Complete surgical resection remains the most effective treatment for patients with early-stage non-small cell lung cancer (NSCLC), provided they have been adequately staged and are medically operable. Under these conditions a 5-year survival rate of 60–75% for patients with stage I disease and 40–50% for patients with stage II can be expected. Similar survival data using the revised TNM staging system were recently reported by the Japanese.[1] After analyzing 3043 resectable lung cancer cases, the 5-year survival rate for patients with stage II disease was 57–45% and that for patients with stage II was 45–57%.

Surgery alone

While complete surgical resection is undeniably the standard of care, the technique to achieve a complete resection is debatable, with the advent of minimally invasive surgery (Table 7.1). Solaini et al[2] published their experience with VATS (video-assisted thoracic surgery) lobectomies in 87 lung cancer patients and 38 patients with benign lesions or solitary metastases. The procedure was considered safe, with a postoperative complication rate of 12% and a median postoperative stay of 5.8 days. For patients with stage I NSCLC, the 3-year survival rate was 90%. Nomori et al[3] conducted a retrospective comparison of VATS lobectomy with ALT (anterior limited thoracotomy) lobectomy in lung cancer. In each group, 33 cases were reviewed. The patients in the VATS group initially experienced less postoperative pain requiring less analgesia, but by week 2 no difference in pain was apparent between the two groups. Other factors, including number of lymph nodes sampled, operating time, blood loss, chest tube drainage, and pulmonary function, were similar between the groups. VATS lobectomy is especially attractive for the elderly population. Koizumi et al[4] reviewed the charts from 87 elderly patients undergoing resection for peripheral stage I NSCLC. Of these patients, 52 had a VATS lobectomy and 35 underwent a standard lobectomy. The 5-year survival rates were 60% and 54%, respectively. These three articles support the use of

Table 7.1 Treatment of resectable NSCLC with surgery alone

Authors	Stage	No. of patients	Treatment[a]	Results
Solaini et al[2]	N0	87	VATS lobectomy	3-yr survival rate 90%
Nomori et al[3]	N0	33	VATS lobectomy	No difference in
		33	ALT lobectomy	parameters evaluated
Koizumi et al[4]	N0	52	VATS lobectomy	5-yr survival rate 60%
		35	Standard lobectomy	5-yr survival rate 54%
Okada et al[5]	N0	70	Segmentectomy	5-yr survival rate 87%
		139	Lobectomy	5-yr survival rate 88%
Miller et al[6]	N0	75	Lobectomy	5-yr survival rate 92%
		25	Limited resection	5-yr survival rate 47%
Wu et al[9]	N0–N2	160	Radical lymphadenectomy	5-yr survival rate (stage I) 81% ($p < 0.014$)
		160	Conventional lymphadenectomy	5-yr survival rate (stage I) 59%
				No survival difference II or IIIA
Elia et al[11]	N0–N2	57	Extrapleural resection	No survival difference
		47	En bloc resection	
Magdeleinat et al[12]	N0–N2	79	Extrapleural resection	No survival difference
		122	En bloc resection	
Facciolo et al[13]	N0–N2	104	En bloc resection	5-yr survival rate 61%

[a] VATS, video-assisted thoracic surgery; ALT, anterior limited thoracotomy.

VATS lobectomy for lung cancer, but randomized trials need to be conducted expeditiously to draw a definitive conclusion about VATS lobectomy as a curative cancer operation.

With the increased detection rate of small tumors, the extent of surgical resection has reemerged as a controversial issue (Table 7.1). Okada et al[5] prospectively enrolled 70 patients with cT1 (<2 cm) tumors into a trial of segmentectomy with lymph node dissection, and compared the results with 139 historical controls undergoing lobectomy. The 5-year survival rate was 87% for extended segmentectomy and 88% for lobectomy. No patient in the segmentectomy group developed a local recurrence. Miller et al[6] reviewed the records of 100 patients with tumors 1 cm or smaller. Of these patients, 75 underwent lobectomy and 25 had a limited resection – either a segmentectomy (n = 12) or a wedge resection (n = 13). They reported that survival was impacted by the operative procedure but not by patient characteristics. Typically, poorer-risk patients have a lesser operation, but in this analysis the patient characteristics were similar between the two groups. The 5-year lung cancer-specific rate in patients with lobectomy was 92% versus 47% after limited resection (p = 0.07). However, the 5-year lung cancer-specific rates were similar between lobectomy and segmentectomy (92% versus 75%). Local recurrence rates were not statistically different (13% for lobectomy, 8% for segmentectomy, and 31% for wedge resection). The authors maintain that lobectomy with lymph node dissection is the preferred operation but that segmentectomy should be further explored.

A pivotal question surrounding the extent of surgical resection required is the relationship between tumor size and nodal metastases. Ohta et al[7] examined 3081 lymph nodes from 181 patients with peripheral stage I NSCLC who had undergone complete resection. The majority of patients had adenocarcinoma (n = 155) and a few patients had squamous histology (n = 26). Nodal micrometastases were detected in 44 patients (24%). There was no difference in tumor size between the node-positive and node-negative adenocarcinoma groups (2.2 cm and 2.1 cm, respectively). Nodal metastasis was found in 19 of 95 (20%) patients with adenocarcinomas of 1.1–2.0 cm, and 4 of 11 (36%) patients had positive nodes with a primary tumor size of 1 cm or less. Tumor size was influential in the small subset of patients with squamous cell carcinoma. The mean tumor size in node-positive patients was 4.8 cm, versus 3.2 cm in node-negative patients. No patient with a tumor size of 2 cm or less had evidence of nodal involvement. Immunohistochemical evaluation for vascular endothelial growth factor (VEGF) was also assessed. Patients with nodal micrometastasis and VEGF overexpression had poorer survival times, while node-positive, VEGF-negative patients had survival times comparable to those of node-negative patients. Another study reviewed nodal status of patients with peripheral tumors of 2 cm or less.[8] Among the 170 patients with adenocarcinoma, 38 (22%) had hilar or mediastinal metastases, but no nodal disease was detected in tumors that were 1 cm or smaller (16 patients). None of the 20 patients with squamous cell carcinoma had nodal metastases. These studies suggest that tumor size is an unpredictable indicator of nodal metastasis in adenocarcinoma but may have value in patients with squamous cell histology.

Lymph node dissection is not only valuable for determining the extent of disease but is also therapeutic. However, the literature has not clearly shown a survival impact for radical mediastinal lymphadenectomy. A recent analysis by Wu et al[9] provides additional insight into this controversy (Table 7.1). They randomly divided 320 patients with stage I–IIIA NSCLC into two groups: radical lymphadenectomy (RL) or conventional lymphadenectomy (CL). Each group enrolled 160 patients. The mean numbers of lymph nodes dissected were 9.5 versus 3.6, respectively. No difference in overall survival was observed in patients with stage II or IIIA disease, but in patients with stage I disease the 5-year survival rate was 81% for the RL group and 59% ($p < 0.014$) for the CL group. In a multivariate analysis of all patients, the postoperative TNM stage, metastasis ratio of lymph nodes, and extent of lymphadenectomy influenced long-term survival. The investigators concluded that systematic mediastinal lymphadenectomy is preferred. Sagawa et al[10] suggest that a complete systemic nodal dissection can be accomplished by VATS. In this study, 29 patients with stage I NSCLC prospectively underwent VATS lobectomy and mediastinal dissection. The average number of lymph nodes resected was 40 for right-sided tumors and 37 for left-sided tumors. Whether this translates into improved survival rates compared to those of conventional sampling is unknown.

Two surgical approaches are used to resected tumors invading the chest wall: extrapleural resection and en bloc resection (Table 7.1). Elia et al[11] retrospectively assessed 110 patients with tumors involving the chest wall. No significant survival difference was noted between the 57 patients undergoing an extrapleural resection and the 47 having an en bloc resection. Survival was dependent on the presence or absence of nodal disease. A second retrospective study by Magdeleinat et al[12] of 201 cases concurs with these results, showing that both surgical techniques are feasible to obtain a complete resection. This study also showed that the depth of invasion into the chest wall and nodal involvement independently affected survival. Finally, Facciolo et al[13] retrospectively reviewed the charts from 104 patients undergoing en bloc resection. The overall 5-year survival rate was 61%. Nodal disease and depth of invasion into the chest wall influenced outcome, with 5-year survival rates of 79% for patients with pleural extension versus 54% for patients with soft tissue and bone extension ($p = 0.014$).

The optimal treatment for medically inoperable patients with early-stage NSCLC is undefined. Traditionally, radiotherapy has been offered to these patients. McGarry et al[14] retrospectively reviewed the survival data on 149 male veterans with stage I and IIA NSCLC from 1994 to 1999. Of these patients, 49 received no cancer therapy, 36 received radiotherapy, and 43 underwent surgical resection. The median survival times were 14 months, 20 months, and 46 months, respectively. The average tumor size was 3 cm in the no-therapy group, 4 cm in the radiotherapy group, and 3 cm in the surgical group. The majority of patients treated with thoracic radiation received palliative doses for symptom control (n = 23). The 13 patients who received curative doses survived 5 months longer. These results reconfirm that surgical resection is the only curative therapy for early-stage NSCLC.

To minimize radiation toxicity, stereotactic radiotherapy (SRT) is under investigation. In a study by Uematsu et al,[15] 50 patients with stage I NSCLC, including 21 medically inoperable patients and 18 previously radiated patients, received 50–60 Gy in 5–10 fractions for 1–2 weeks via the stereotactic approach. The 3-year survival rate was 66%, with 6 patients dying from disease. No adverse effects were observed. Supporting the utility of SRT, Gilson et al[16] administered SRT (180–1000 Gy in 3–8 fractions) to 202 pretreated patients with primary lung cancer. They reported an 88% control rate (defined as cessation of tumor growth or shrinkage or disappearance of the tumor) and the treatment was well tolerated. An alternative novel technique is radiofrequency ablation (RFA). Kang et al[17] reported on the use of RFA in 20 patients: 8 with primary lung cancer and 12 with lung metastases from breast or colon cancer. Treatment times were between 5 and 15 minutes to achieve a power run of 999, which was maintained for 2 minutes. Positron emission tomography (PET) scans pre and post treatment were used to assess response. Kang et al found that the benefit of RFA was limited to tumors of 3.5 cm or smaller. Toxicities were mild, with 6 patients developing fevers, but 5 patients did develop a pneumothorax from the procedure. SRT and RFA may be an effective alternative with less toxicity for medically inoperable patients and patients with localized recurrence. More studies are planned.

Adjuvant therapies

Several recent reviews of adjuvant therapies in early NSCLC all conclude that there is no convincing evidence that any therapy in the adjuvant setting consistently improves survival.[18–20] In 2001, three small randomized trials reported their results administering adjuvant therapy (Table 7.2). Trodella et al[21] gave adjuvant radiotherapy to 104 pathologic stage I NSCLC patients. Local recurrence occurred in 2.2% of patients receiving radiotherapy versus 23% in the observation arm. Disease-free survivals were 71% and 60%, respectively (p = 0.039), with 5-year overall survival rates of 67% for the radiotherapy arm and 58% for the control arm (p = 0.048). Acute radiation toxicity was mild; 19 patients developed radiographic evidence of fibrosis, but only 1 patient was symptomatic. The second trial, from China, administered adjuvant chemotherapy consisting of cyclophosphamide, vincristine, doxorubicin, and lomustine (CCNA) for four cycles or observation to 70 patients with stage I–III NSCLC.[22] The overall 5-year survival rates were 49% for the chemotherapy group and 31% for the surgery alone group, which were not statistically different. For patients with stage III disease, adjuvant chemotherapy was associated with a significant prolongation in survival (44% versus 21%; p = 0.025). The last small randomized trial, conducted in Italy, included only patients with stage IB disease.[23] In this trial, 33 patients were registered to the adjuvant

Table 7.2　Adjuvant therapy for resectable NSCLC

Authors	Stage	No. of patients	Treatment[a]	5-year survival rate (%)
Trodella et al[21]	N0	51	RT	67　($p = 0.048$)
		53	Observation	58
Xu et al[22]	N0–N2	35	CT	49
		35	Observation	31
Mineo et al[23]	N0	33	CT	59　($p = 0.04$)
		33	Observation	30
Kato et al[24]	N0	202	Ubenimex	81　($p = 0.02$)
		198	Placebo	74
Sakamoto et al[25]	N0–N2	1520	CT + OK-432	51　($p = 0.001$)
			CT + placebo	44
Landareneau et al[26]	N0	60	^{125}I brachytherapy	68　(at 31 months)
Ichinose et al[36]	N2	59	CT	49⎫(at 3 years)
		60	Observation	49⎭

[a] RT, radiotherapy; CT, chemotherapy.

chemotherapy arm, which consisted of cisplatin (100 mg/m^2 on day 1) with etoposide (120 mg/m^2 on days 1–3) for six cycles and 33 patients were observed. With a minimum follow-up of 5 years, local recurrence rates were 24% for the surgery-alone arm and 18% with adjuvant chemotherapy. Distant metastases developed in 43% and 30%, respectively. The 5-year survival rate was 59% for the adjuvant group, compared with 30% for the no-adjuvant-therapy group ($p = 0.04$).

Although these small trials suggest a benefit for adjuvant therapy, large randomized trials do not. In 2001, no data from a phase III adjuvant trial were presented. Thus, we continue to await the results from seven randomized trials evaluating adjuvant chemotherapy, including trials with newer cytotoxic agents. Five trials have been completed and two are ongoing.

An old adjuvant strategy is immunotherapy. Kato et al[24] conducted a randomized phase III trial of the immunomodulator ubenimex in 400 patients with pathologic stage I squamous cell carcinoma. Ubenimex was administered orally 30 mg/day for 2 years versus placebo. The 5-year survival rate was 81% for ubenimex versus 74% for placebo ($p = 0.02$), and the disease-free survival rate was also superior for the ubenimex group (72% versus 62%; $p = 0.02$). No differences in toxicities were observed, except for increased anorexia with ubenimex. Overall, there was a survival benefit for ubenimex, but a confirmatory trial should be performed. Recently a meta-analysis of adjuvant immunochemotherapy with OK-432 (a penicillin-treated, lyophilized preparation of *Streptococcus pyogenes*) from Japan provides provocative results.[25] Eleven randomized trials of chemotherapy with or without OK-432 conducted before 1991 in 1520 cases of resectable NSCLC were analyzed. The 5-year survival rates for eligible patients were 51% for the immunochemotherapy group and 44% for the chemotherapy-alone group ($p = 0.001$). A subset of four trials with central randomization produced a significantly longer survival time for patients receiving additional immunotherapy ($p = 0.049$). These data support the investigation of newer immunotherapy strategies such as vaccines.

Meanwhile, an exciting adjuvant trial evaluating the oral epidermal growth factor receptor (EGFR) small-molecule inhibitor ZD1839 is being launched by the Canadian National Cancer Institute (NCI) with the USA as a participant. Patients with stage I, II, and IIIA (N0–1) NSCLC who have undergone a curative resection will be randomized to ZD1839 or placebo for 2 years.

The role of adjuvant radiotherapy has also produced disappointing results after lobectomy for early-stage lung cancer, but its value in decreasing local recurrence after limited resection is an uncharted arena that deserves investigation. One recent trial has yet to report efficacy data, but stated that compliance with treatment was poor, opening the door for alternative approaches such as brachytherapy. Landareneau et al[26] administered intraoperative ^{125}I brachytherapy to 60 patients with stage I NSCLC undergoing wedge resection or segmentectomy (Table 7.2). After placement of a ^{125}I mesh along the staple line, a dose of 10 000–12 000 cGy was given. The local recurrence rate was 0 of 58 patients, which is superior to the 17% local recurrence rate reported in historical series. Distant metastases developed in 15 patients. Importantly, pulmonary function was not affected. At a mean of 31 months, 68% of patients remain alive. This encouraging result should be pursued in a larger study.

Neoadjuvant therapy

A detailed review of neoadjuvant chemotherapy in early-stage NSCLC by Depierre and Westeel[27] discusses the past trials and provides a schema of seven large randomized trials comparing preoperative chemotherapy plus surgery verses surgery alone that are planned or ongoing throughout the world. Only one pilot trial reported results of preoperative chemotherapy in early-stage NSCLC. The North Central Cancer Treatment Group (NCCTG) treated 52 mediastinoscopy-negative patients with three cycles of paclitaxel (200 mg/m²) with carboplatin (AUC 7.5).[28] An objective response to chemotherapy was achieved in 59% of the patients. Complete resections were accomplished in 36 of 46 patients (78%). With a median follow-up of 22 months, the 2-year survival rate was 73%. The major toxicity from chemotherapy was grade 3/4 neutropenia, which occurred in 23 patients.

Four publications reported on the influence of preoperative chemotherapy on surgical resection. Breton et al[29] examined the postoperative complication rate from a large French randomized trial comparing two cycles of neoadjuvant MIP (mitomycin, ifosfamide, and cisplatin) versus resection alone in patients with stage IB–IIIA NSCLC. The total number of complications was 39 versus 27 ($p = 0.12$), respectively, with 49% versus 36% ($p = 0.34$) of these patients dying from their complications. Martin et al[30] retrospectively reviewed the Memorial Sloan-Kettering experience with neoadjuvant chemotherapy from 1993 to 1999. This review included 470 patients with stage I–IV NSCLC receiving a variety of regimens, but primarily MVP (mitomycin, vinblastine, and cisplatin) and PC (paclitaxel and carboplatin). A minority of patients received radiotherapy. The major complication rate was acceptable at 27%. The total mortality rates were 2.4% for lobectomies and 11.3% for pneumonectomies. Preoperative chemotherapy was not found to be a risk factor for morbidity or mortality in the multivariate analysis. In contrast, colleagues from Vanderbilt reported an increase in morbidity with neoadjuvant therapy.[31] This single-institution experience from 1997 to 1999 included 34 patients with early-stage disease (IB–IIIA, N0–1) receiving paclitaxel and carboplatin for three cycles compared with 67 patients undergoing resection without prior chemotherapy compared to no systemic therapy. They observed significant increases in life-threatening complications (27% versus 3%), major complications (47% versus 19%), reintubation (18% versus 3%), and tracheostomy (0% versus 12%) in patients receiving chemotherapy. No hospital mortality was observed. The last study, conducted in Spain, was a case–control study examining postoperative morbidity and mortality in 42 patients receiving induction chemotherapy compared with 42 matched controls undergoing surgery alone.[32] No postoperative mortality was recorded. The total morbidity rate was 26% with chemotherapy versus 43% in controls ($p = 0.08$), suggesting no significant influence of chemotherapy on postoperative complication rates. Overall, preoperative chemotherapy does not increase surgical complications.

POTENTIALLY RESECTABLE STAGE III NSCLC

For patients with completely resected stage III (N2) disease, the role of additional therapy is ill defined owing to the heterogeneity in the stage and the small number of patients receiving surgery alone. Ichinose et al[33] attempted to identify risk factors for recurrence and survival in 406 patients with resected N2 NSCLC that might allow selection of patients who should have adjuvant therapy. In the multivariate analysis, survival was worse in patients with multiple N2 stations, pathologic T2, T3, or N1 disease, and age older than 65. Local recurrence was increased with multiple N2 lymph nodes and clinical N1 or N2 disease. Patients with multiple involved mediastinal lymph nodes had a 5-year survival rate of 17% and a freedom from local recurrence rate of 48%, compared with 43% and 75%, respectively, for patients with an isolated mediastinal lymph node. Ichinose et al surmised that the number of mediastinal lymph nodes involved is an important prognostic factor.

Bueno et al[34] retrospectively reviewed medical records of 103 N2 patients who received a variety of induction regimens followed by surgical resection, and demonstrated that eradication of tumor in the mediastinum had a 5-year survival rate of 36%, compared with 9% for patients with persistent tumor in hilar or mediastinal lymph nodes. These data are consistent with previous data reported by the Southwest Oncology Group (SWOG) showing an impressive 6-year survival rate of 33% for stage III patients with a complete pathologic response in the mediastinum after concurrent chemoradiation followed by surgery.[35]

Adjuvant therapies

The Japan Clinical Oncology Group (JCOG) presented data in 2001 on their randomized phase III trial of adjuvant cisplatin (80 mg/m^2 on day 1) with vindesine (3 mg/m^2 on days 1 and 8) every 4 weeks for three cycles versus no treatment (Table 7.2).[36] This trial enrolled 119 completely resected pIIIA (N2) patients. The median survival times were 35.5 months in the chemotherapy arm and 35.2 months in the no-treatment group. The 3-year survival rates for both arms were 49%. The Germans also presented information from a randomized trial of adjuvant radiotherapy (50 Gy in 5 weeks) versus adjuvant chemotherapy (cisplatin 75 mg/m^2 on day 1 plus ifosfamide 1.5 g/m^2 on days 1–4 every 4 weeks for three cycles) followed by the same radiotherapy in patients with resectable N2 disease.[37] The trial was designed to show a 6-month improvement in survival with chemotherapy. Owing to slow accrual the trial was stopped after 150 patients. The median survival for all patients was 34 months, with a 3-year survival rate of 46%. No survival differences were observed between the two groups. Greco et al[38] conducted a phase II trial to evaluate the feasibility and toxicity of adjuvant paclitaxel and carboplatin alone or with radiotherapy for patients with resected stage IB–IV NSCLC. Patients with stage IB disease received only adjuvant chemotherapy, while all other patients received subsequent concurrent chemoradiotherapy. Ninety percent of patients (92 of 102) received all three cycles of paclitaxel and carboplatin, while 73% of patients (49 of 67) received the additional full doses of concurrent therapy. Therapy was well tolerated. While survival data were premature, the feasibility of delivering adjuvant therapy is important for the small subset of patients who are upstaged from their surgical resection.

Despite the lack of clinical data, most physicians would recommend adjuvant therapy for resected stage III (N2) disease, but the modality offered is highly variable and depends on patient and tumor characteristics. Modalities recommended include radiotherapy, chemotherapy, or both. Furthermore, it is unlikely that trials to evaluate adjuvant therapy after curative resection will be designed, because of the popularity of neoadjuvant regimens.

Neoadjuvant therapies

Eberhardt et al[39] published a comprehensive review of the current status of preoperative therapy for stage III NSCLC, citing the three well-known small randomized trials by Rosell, Roth, and Pass favoring preoperative chemotherapy prior to surgical resection for patients with N2 disease. They also discussed eight phase II trials of induction chemoradiotherapy prior to resection. Overall, these trials reported a high frequency of preoperative downstaging, resulting in an increase in complete resection rates. However, pathologic complete responses remain low at 15–25%, necessitating new studies. Schemas for ongoing or recently completed phase III trials were displayed.

New data from four small studies were published in 2001 (Table 7.3). Spasova et al[40] gave induction vinorelbine and cisplatin to 56 patients with marginally resectable or unresectable stage III patients. Thirty-two percent of patients were able to undergo complete resections. Postoperative complications were rare and no treatment-related deaths were reported. With a minimal follow-up of 24 months, patients who were completely resected had the most favorable outcome. Three studies administered gemcitabine plus cisplatin as neoadjuvant treatment. Santo et al[41] administered three cycles of gemcitabine/cisplatin to 43 patients with stage IIIA (N2) and IIIB NSCLC. Twenty-six patients (67%) had an objective response to induction chemotherapy and 8 had stable disease. A complete resection was achieved in 13 of 16 patients (81%). The remaining 18 patients received radiation. Yang et al[42] also administered three cycles of gemcitabine and cisplatin to 52 stage III patients. The overall response rate was similar at 64%. Thirty-six patients were operable, but only 35% were able to have a complete resection. The median survival was 19.1 months with a 2 year survival rate of 34%. The third trial gave preoperative gemcitabine plus cisplatin to 36 patients with proven N2 disease.[43] Twenty-five patients (70%) had a partial response to chemotherapy and were surgically explored. Eighteen complete resections (70%) were accomplished.

Table 7.3 Neoadjuvant treatment for stage III NSCLC

Authors	Stage	No. of patients	Treatment[a]	Response rate (%)[b]	Median survival (months)[b]	Long-term survival (years)[b]
Spasova et al[40]	IIIA/B	56	CT	NR	NR	NR
Santo et al[41]	IIIA/B	43	CT	67	NR	NR
Yang et al[42]	IIIA/B	52	CT	64	19.1	34% (2)
Voltolini et al[43]	IIIA	36	CT	70	21 (surgical group) 8 (nonsurgical group)	20% (3); 30% (3) surgical group
Weitberg et al[44]	IIIA	33	CT and RT	NR	NR	42% DFS (12)
Wright et al[45]	IIIA/B	20	RT	35	NR	49% (4)
		15	CT and RT	87	NR	84% (4) p = (0.01)
Raefsky et al[46]	II/III	61	CT and RT	54	NR	37% (2); 43% (2) surgical group
Ahn et al[47]	IIIA	31	CT and RT	NR	19	

[a] CT, chemotherapy; RT, radiotherapy.
[b] NR, not reported

The median survival for the surgical group was 21 months. The overall 3 year survival was 20% for all patients and 30% for the surgical subgroup compared to 8 months for the nonsurgical group. These trials suggest that induction gemcitabine/cisplatin produces high response rates and encouraging resection rates, and support its use in several randomized trials.

If chemotherapy is tolerable and does not increase operative risk, what is the role of neoadjuvant chemoradiotherapy (Table 7.3)? Weitberg et al[44] reported a 42% disease-specific survival rate with 12 years of follow-up in 33 patients receiving cisplatin and etoposide plus thoracic radiation (60 Gy) followed by surgery. Wright et al[45] conducted a retrospective study on 35 patients who underwent induction chemoradiotherapy or radiotherapy for superior sulcus tumors. All patients had T3 or T4 disease but none had N2 involvement. Fifteen patients had bimodality induction therapy and 14 were able to undergo a complete resection (93%), as compared with 16 of 20 patients (80%) receiving only induction radiation. Impressively, 13 of 15 patients (87%) undergoing chemoradiation followed by surgery had pathological complete responses (CRs) or near CRs, as compared with 7 of 20 patients (35%) treated with radiation followed by surgery. As expected, the 4-year overall survival rate was superior for the trimodality group at 84% versus 49% ($p = 0.01$) for the bimodality group, and the local recurrence rate was 0% versus 30%, respectively ($p = 0.02$). A pilot trial of weekly paclitaxel 50 mg/m^2 plus carboplatin AUC 2 with concurrent radiotherapy (45 Gy) was conducted at the Minnie Pearl Cancer Network.[46] In this trial, 61 patients primarily with stage IIIA or B NSCLC received this therapy and 54 patients completed the regimen. A clinical response was achieved in 54%. Twenty-nine patients proceeded to surgery, 28 patients had a complete resection, and 12 had pathologic CRs. The remaining 32 patients received additional chemoradiotherapy. This regimen of concurrent chemoradiotherapy was feasible, highly active, and well tolerated prior to surgery. One additional small prospective trial from Korea administered 45 Gy of thoracic radiation with two cycles of cisplatin and etoposide.[47] Of the 31 patients entered, 23 patients completed the trimodality schema. Complete resections were accomplished in 22 (71%), pathological CRs in 14%, and downstaging in 68%. The median survival for the 22 resected patients was 19 months, with a 2-year survival rate of 43%, compared with 19 months and 37%, respectively, for the entire group. Fifty-eight percent of the patients experienced moderate to severe esophagitis. These results are comparable to those of other small series. The role of neoadjuvant chemoradiotherapy awaits the results from the US Intergroup trial assessing trimodality therapy (chemoradiotherapy followed by surgery) versus bimodality therapy (chemoradiotherapy) in N2 patients. Preliminary data are expected in 2003.

One article addressed patterns of relapse in patients with N2 disease who received preoperative cisplatin-based chemotherapy followed by surgery.[48] Eighty-one patients receiving bimodality treatment were compared with 186 patients who received surgery alone. Distant metastases developed in 28% of patients versus 38% of patients, respectively. With a median follow-up of 52 months, the 2- and 5-year survival rates for the chemotherapy group were 35%

and 17%, as compared with 26% and 9% for the surgery-alone group. Preoperative chemotherapy was associated with a better prognosis in a multivariate analysis ($p = 0.001$). Interestingly, more brain metastases occurred in the chemotherapy-treated group, which was significant in the multivariate analysis along with adenocarcinoma histology ($p < 0.05$). This phenomenon has been observed in several studies, and suggests that prophylactic brain irradiation should be reconsidered.

UNRESECTABLE STAGE III NSCLC

Combined-modality treatment

The approach to the management of locally advanced, unresectable NSCLC has evolved over the years from a radiotherapy-alone strategy to a sequential approach with induction chemotherapy followed by radiotherapy. More recently, a concurrent chemoradiotherapy approach has advanced as the standard of care in the USA. The addition of chemotherapy during radiotherapy appears to enhance local/regional control as well as reducing micrometastatic spread. The majority of drugs used in the treatment of NSCLC have been found to enhance the cytotoxic effects of radiation. Concomitant administration of chemotherapy along with radiation may improve the local control by eradicating cells that are resistant to radiation therapy (cells in S phase and hypoxic cells), inhibiting the repair of potentially lethal or sublethal damage, or potentiating the effects of radiation through the accumulation of cells in G_2/M phase (a phase during which cancer cells have enhanced sensitivity to radiation-induced cell kill). The efficacy of concurrent chemoradiation has been confirmed in several meta-analyses of randomized trials comparing radiotherapy alone versus chemotherapy plus radiotherapy, which showed that the combined therapy was superior.[49,50] The greatest differences were reported in trials employing cisplatin-based chemotherapy regimens. There were numerous ways in which the modalities were combined, including sequential chemotherapy followed by radiotherapy, concurrent chemotherapy and radiotherapy, and alternating chemotherapy and radiotherapy. There were few differences among these approaches in the meta-analyses. More recent results from two randomized trials evaluating sequential versus concurrent chemotherapy both demonstrated more favorable outcomes with a concurrent approach. Thus, concurrent chemoradiotherapy is the standard of care for the treatment of locally advanced NSCLC.[51,52] Yet to be defined are the optimal volume, dose, schedule, and fractionation of radiotherapy. These issues are currently under investigation in several Radiation Therapy Oncology Group (RTOG)-sponsored clinical trials. In addition, clinical trials in locally advanced NSCLC are evaluating various combinations and sequencing of chemotherapy doublets in induction, consolidation, and concurrent settings to try and improve the therapeutic index (improved tumor control/reduced toxicity). Below, we review some of the important randomized and selected non-randomized trials reported in 2001 that may help to answer some of these questions.

Randomized phase II–III trials

Defining the optimal timing and administration of chemotherapy with radiation remains a dynamic process. In an attempt to clarify this issue, Curran et al[53] recently reported the results of a randomized, multi-institutional phase II study of three different chemoradiotherapy regimens administered for the treatment of locally advanced NSCLC (Table 7.4). The findings were compared with the best arm of RTOG 88-08 (median survival 13.7 months). This locally advanced multimodality protocol (LAMP) compared a regimen consisting of induction therapy with carboplatin/paclitaxel and concurrent carboplatin/paclitaxel and thoracic radiation (arm B) versus a regimen of sequential carboplatin/paclitaxel and radiation (arm A) or concurrent carboplatin/paclitaxel and radiation followed by consolidative carboplatin/paclitaxel (arm C). The results at interim analysis indicated an inferior outcome in arm B, with a median survival of 11 months. In this arm, 17% of the patients were unable to receive the planned concurrent treatment, suggesting that the induction phase was too intense, compromising delivery of concurrent chemotherapy and radiation.

To evaluate newer combinations with cisplatin, the Cancer and Leukemia Group B (CALGB) reported preliminary results in 2001 of a randomized phase II study (CALGB 9431) of two cycles of induction chemotherapy followed by two additional cycles of the same drugs with concomitant radiotherapy (Table 7.4).[54] Eligible patients received four cycles of cisplatin at 80 mg/m^2 on days 1, 22, 43, and 64 with: (arm 1) gemcitabine 1250 mg/m^2 (days 1, 8, 22, and 29) and 600 mg/m^2 (days 43, 50, 64, and 71); (arm 2) paclitaxel 225 mg/m^2 for 3 hours (days 1 and 22) and 135 mg/m^2 (days 43 and 64); or (arm 3) vinorelbine 25 mg/m^2 (days 1, 8, 15, 22, and 29) and 15 mg/m^2 (days 43, 50, 64, and 71). Radiotherapy was initiated on day 43 at 2 Gy/day (total dose 66 Gy). Similar response rates after completion of chemoradiation in the 175 eligible patients analyzed for this study were observed in the three arms: 74%, 67%, and 73% respectively. The median survival for all patients was 17 months. The 3-year survival rates for the patients on the three arms were 28%, 19%, and 23%, respectively. Not surprisingly, toxicities during induction chemotherapy consisted primarily of grade 3 or 4 granulocytopenia. Grade 3 or 4 toxicities during concomitant chemoradiotherapy consisted of thrombocytopenia, granulocytopenia, and esophagitis. The cohort receiving cisplatin and vinorelbine had only a 27% incidence of granulocytopenia, in contrast to the 48–51% seen in the other cohorts. Additionally, grade 3/4 esophagitis was lower in the vinorelbine group (24% versus 38–58% in the other groups).

A secondary analysis of RTOG 94-10 examined the outcomes in elderly patients versus younger patients treated in a phase III trial comparing concurrent chemoradiotherapy versus sequential chemoradiotherapy.[55] Chemotherapy consisted of cisplatin (100 mg/m^2 on days 1 and 29) and vinblastine (5 mg/m^2 weekly × 5). An additional experimental arm evaluated twice-daily radiation with concur-

Table 7.4   Randomized phase III trials of combined-modality studies in unresectable stage III NSCLC

Authors	Treatment[a]	No. of patients	Response rate (%)[b]	Survival	Toxicity grade 3/4
Curran et al[53]	Carboplatin/paclitaxel → RT (A); Carboplatin/paclitaxel → Carboplatin/paclitaxel/RT (B); Carboplatin/paclitaxel/RT → Carboplatin/paclitaxel (C)	243 randomized	NR	Arm B had an inferior median survival of 11 months	*Arm B* Hematologic 25% Esophagitis 18% Non-hematologic 8%
Vokes[54]	Cisplatin/gemcitabine → Cisplatin/gemcitabine/RT (1)	62	74	28% (3-year)	*Induction:* Granulocytopenia 48–55%
	Cisplatin/paclitaxel → Cisplatin/paclitaxel/RT (2)	58	67	19% (3-year)	*Concurrent:* Thrombocytopenia 53%, 6%, and 0% in arms 1, 2, and 3, respectively
	Cisplatin/vinorelbine → Cisplatin/vinorelbine/RT (3)	55	73	23% (3-year)	Granulocytopenia 51%, 48%, and 27% in arms 1, 2, and 3, respectively Esophagitis 50%, 38%, and 24% in arms 1, 2, and 3, respectively

[a] RT, radiotherapy.
[b] NR, not reported.

rent cisplatin plus oral etoposide. Although the incidence of acute esophagitis was higher in patients older than 70, in both the sequential and concurrent groups, the median survival favored concurrent chemoradiation (22.4 months) over sequential chemoradiation (16.4 months). The median survival for patients younger than 70 was similar in the concurrent and sequential chemoradiotherapy arms (15.5 and 16.0 months, respectively).

The use of chemoradiation for treatment of locally advanced NSCLC may incur significant toxicity in the form of esophagitis and radiation-induced pneumonitis. Developing ways of reducing radiation-induced toxicity is critical to improve the therapeutic gain for patients with inoperable NSCLC. In this regard, a phase III trial was conducted to determine the efficacy of amifostine, a thiol compound, to reduce the severity of pulmonary and esophageal morbidity in patients undergoing concurrent chemoradiation.[56] This trial enrolled 62 patients from 1997 to 2001. At the time of this report, a median follow-up of 6 months demonstrated a significant reduction in acute esophagitis from 26% in the control group to 6.5% in the group receiving intravenous amifostine (500 mg twice weekly) ($p = 0.038$). Acute pneumonitis was reduced from 19% to 3.2% in the group receiving amifostine ($p = 0.045$).

Non-randomized trials

Newer chemotherapy regimens given concurrently with chest radiotherapy have been investigated in phase I and II trials. Paclitaxel plus carboplatin has emerged as a popular regimen for the treatment of metastatic NSCLC because it is efficacious with milder toxicity than a cisplatin-containing regimen. Both paclitaxel and carboplatin are radiosensitizers and have also been used extensively in the USA on a weekly schedule with thoracic radiotherapy. Additional support for this regimen continues to grow. Guichard et al[57] enrolled 51 patients in a phase II trial from 1998 to 2000 that administered weekly paclitaxel at 40 mg/m^2 with weekly carboplatin (AUC 2) in conjunction with radiotherapy to a dose of 65 Gy in patients with stage III NSCLC. Of the 31 evaluable patients, 28 were men and 22 of 34 patients presented with stage IIIB disease. At a median follow-up of 15 months, the regimen was well tolerated, and the 18-month disease-free and overall survival rates were 52% and 63%, respectively.

A popular strategy has also been to give newer chemotherapy agents prior to or after concurrent therapy (Table 7.5). A Swedish study evaluated response rates in patients with stage III NSCLC receiving induction carboplatin/paclitaxel for three cycles followed by weekly paclitaxel (60 mg/m^2) and carboplatin (AUC 2) and concurrent thoracic radiation (60 Gy in 6 weeks).[58] The study enrolled 53 patients from 1999 to 2000; the majority (40) were stage IIIB. Four grade 3 esophageal toxicities were observed in the initial 42 evaluable patients with an overall response rate of 71%. Finally, Rosenman et al[59] conducted a dose-escalating three-dimensional thoracic radiation trial incorporating two cycles of induction carboplatin (AUC 6) and paclitaxel (225 mg/m^2) followed by weekly carboplatin/paclitaxel combined with radiation. The intent was to determine if

Table 7.5 Phase I–II trials of induction/consolidation chemotherapy with concurrent chemoradiation for unresectable stage II–III NSCLC

Authors	Treatment[a]	No. of patients	Response rate (%)[b,c]	Toxicity grade 3/4[d]	Median survival (months)[b]
Sirzen et al[58]	Induction carboplatin/paclitaxel ×3 / Weekly carboplatin/paclitaxel + RT (60 Gy)	53	71	Grade 3 esophagitis 12% (4 patients)	NR
Rosenman et al[59]	Induction carboplatin/paclitaxel ×2 / Weekly carboplatin/paclitaxel + RT (60 Gy) / Consolidation carboplatin/paclitaxel	62	52	Esophagitis 8%	24
Lau et al[60]	Weekly carboplatin/paclitaxel + RT (60 Gy)	34	71	Esophagitis 38% / Neutropenia 12%	17
George et al[61]	Induction carboplatin/paclitaxel/irinotecan ×2 / Weekly carboplatin/paclitaxel/irinotecan + RT (66 Gy)	10	NR	Neutropenia main problem, carboplatin dropped	NR
Sakai et al[63]	Carboplatin/docetaxel weekly + RT (60 Gy) / Consolidation carboplatin/docetaxel	23	79	MTD of docetaxel 40 mg/m^2, of C AUC 3	NR
Carabantes et al[65]	Cisplatin/vinorelbine ×3 / Cisplatin/vinorelbine + RT (65–70 Gy) / Non-responders treated with RT alone	28	71 after induction	Anemia 21% / Deep vein chrombosis 7% / Neurologic 11%	NR
Skarin et al[66]	Carboplatin/docetaxel ×2 / Carboplatin/docetaxel + RT (54 Gy) / then S if responder	20	30% after all chemo/RT	Neutropenia	12+

[a] RT, radiotherapy.
[b] NR, not reported.
[c] CR, complete response; PR, partial response.
[d] MTD, maximum tolerated dose.
S, surgery.

delivery of 74 Gy would be feasible. This phase I/II trial enrolled 62 patients, of whom 48 were able to complete the planned treatment course. With a median follow-up of 43 months, the median survival was 24 months, with a 3-year survival rate of 38%; the 3-year survival rate of patients able to complete the trial was 45%. A modest 13% of patients experienced a local regional failure as the only site of failure. Toxicity was reasonable, with only 8% of patients experiencing grade 3/4 esophagitis.

The California Cancer Consortium determined, in a phase II multi-institutional trial, the response and survival rates in patients with stage III NSCLC treated with paclitaxel twice weekly and carboplatin weekly with concurrent thoracic radiotherapy to a dose of 61 Gy.[60] Patients then went on to receive consolidation paclitaxel and carboplatin. In the 34 patients eligible for this study, the overall induction response rate was 71%. At a median follow-up of 20 months, the median survival was 17 months, and the 2-year actuarial survival rate was reported to be 40%.

An effort to add newer radiosensitizers to the carboplatin/paclitaxel regimens has included the administration of irinotecan for patients with unresectable NSCLC.[61] In this regard, a phase I study evaluated the toxicity of induction carboplatin/paclitaxel and irinotecan for two cycles followed by the same regimen with concurrent radiotherapy (66 Gy) in patients with stage III NSCLC. The limiting issue with this regimen was neutropenia with paclitaxel doses of 45 mg/m² and irinotecan at 30 mg/m², requiring a reduction of the paclitaxel dose to 40 mg/m². Carboplatin was subsequently dropped to reduce myelosuppression. The Fox Chase Cancer Center also investigated the addition of dose-escalating weekly irinotecan and weekly cisplatin with thoracic radiation in a phase I study in patients with medically inoperable and surgically unresectable stage II–III NSCLC or locally recurrent NSCLC after resection.[62] Although a small study, approximatly 82% of the 11 evaluable patients were alive at a median follow-up of 13 months. At the time of this report, the maximum-tolerated dose (MTD) of irinotecan had not been reached when combined with fixed-dose cisplatin (25 mg/m²); however, 3 patients experienced grade 3 neutropenia.

Docetaxel has also shown promising activity in NSCLC. Sakai et al[63] evaluated the feasibility of delivering concurrent docetaxel (given twice weekly) with carboplatin and concurrent chest radiotherapy (60 Gy) in patients with stage III NSCLC, followed by consolidative docetaxel/carboplatin. The MTD was docetaxel at 40 mg/m² and carboplatin at an AUC of 3 in the 23 patients entered into this study. In 14 evaluable patients at the time of this report, the response rate was 79%. The Vanderbilt Cancer Center incorporated docetaxel in a weekly regimen combined with thoracic radiation and carboplatin in a phase I trial (15 patients) to determine the MTD and dose-limiting toxicities (DLT) in patients with unresectable stage III NSCLC.[64] Docetaxel was administered weekly for 6 weeks, starting at 20 mg/m². Docetaxel doses were escalated by 10 mg/m² increments in successive cohorts of three patients. DLT was defined as grade 3 or higher non-hematologic and hematologic toxicity using

RTOG toxicity criteria. Once the DLT of docetaxel alone was reached, weekly carboplatin (AUC 2) was added at a DLT-2 dose of docetaxel (i.e. two dose levels below that of DLT). Docetaxel doses were again escalated at 10 mg/m^2 increments in successive cohorts of three new patients to define further DLT and MTD of docetaxel/carboplatin with radiation. Radiation was administered with conventional techniques to the primary tumor and regional lymph nodes (40 Gy), followed by a boost to the tumor (20 Gy). The DLT of weekly docetaxel/radiation was esophagitis and the MTD was 30 mg/m^2 per week for 6 weeks. Nine more patients were added with the concurrent docetaxel/carboplatin and radiation regimen. The DLT of weekly docetaxel/carboplatin with radiation was esophagitis and the MTD of docetaxel was 20 mg/m^2 per week with weekly carboplatin (AUC 2). Evaluating further the response rates with induction chemotherapy followed by concurrent chemoradiotherapy, Carabantes et al[65] entered 28 patients with stage III NSCLC (18 with squamous cell histology) into a phase II trial using cisplatin (100 mg/m^2) and vinorelbine (25 mg/m^2) for three cycles followed by radiotherapy (65–70 Gy) with a 21-day cycle of cisplatin (65 mg/m^2) and vinorelbine (15 mg/m^2). Non-responders received only radiotherapy. Of 28 patients, 22 responded to induction therapy, and neurologic toxicities were most frequent (11%). Skarin et al[66] treated a similar cohort of patients with induction carboplatin and docetaxel followed by concurrent carboplatin/docetaxel (weekly) and radiotherapy (54 Gy). There were 8/20 patients who achieved an objective response-responders in this phase I trial, with neutropenia being the main toxicity.

Gemcitabine is a potent radiosensitizer in preclinical studies; this is partly due to S-phase cell cycle shifts as a result of reduced deoxyadenosine triphosphate pools. Blackstock et al[67] have demonstrated in a phase I trial an MTD of 35 mg/m^2 with twice-weekly gemcitabine with concurrent radiation, resulting in an 88% response rate. Major toxicities included pulmonary fibrosis and esophagitis.

Phase I–III trials with altered-fraction radiotherapy and chemotherapy

To improve upon local regional control rates, many investigators have evaluated the use of altered fractionation techniques (Table 7.6). The rationale is based in part on nullifying the rapid repopulation that can occur in lung cancer. Phase I–III studies have evaluated the utility of delivering twice-daily or three-times daily radiation with chemotherapy. Results of an NCCTG Mayo Clinic phase III study comparing concurrent cisplatin/etoposide and 60 Gy of standard once-daily radiation versus twice-daily radiotherapy (30 Gy in a 20-fraction split course) and concurrent cisplatin/etoposide demonstrated no difference in median or overall survival between the two arms in patients with stage III NSCLC.[68] Of the 234 eligible patients, 123 had stage IIIA disease. The median follow-up was 43 months (range 2–73 months) and the 2-year survival rate was 37% (once-daily radiotherapy) versus 40% (twice-daily radiotherapy). No improvement in local control was observed with the twice-daily radio-

Table 7.6 Phase I–III trials using altered-fraction radiotherapy for patients within unresectable stage II–III NSCLC

Authors	Treatment[a]	No. of patients	Response rate (%)[b]	Toxicity grade 3–4	Survival[b]
Schild et al[68]	Split-course AHRT (60 Gy in 40 fractions) versus daily RT (60 Gy) + cisplatin/etoposide	246 (234 eligible)	NR	Similar in both arms: Esophagitis 18–20% Pneumonitis 11–15% Neutropenia 76–80%	2 year 40% AHRT 37% Daily RT
Jeremic et al[69]	Concurrent carboplatin/etoposide + AHRT (69.6 Gy) ± weekend carboplatin/etoposide	195	NR	Increased hematologic toxicity in weekend chemotherapy group	5-year progression-free survival rate similar, at approximately 27%
Kisohara et al[70]	Concurrent cisplatin/vinorelbine and CBRT (61 Gy in 5 weeks)	27	70%	Neutropenia and leukopenia (78%)	NR
Ohashi et al[71]	Weekly carboplatin/paclitaxel + HRT (69.6 Gy), dose escalation of paclitaxel	15	80%	Lymphocytopenia 100%	NR
Marks et al[72]	Induction carboplatin/paclitaxel or carboplatin/vinorelbine × 2 AHRT dose escalation 73.6–92.8 Gy	36	NR	Two grade 4 toxicities (lung/esophagus) at 86.4 Gy with carboplatin/paclitaxel; RT MTD not reached with carboplatin/vinorelbine up to 86.4 Gy	NR
Schild et al[73]	Daily cisplatin TID RT (57.6 Gy)	20	70%	50% at 7.5 mg/m^2 cisplatin 5/10 pts	16.4 months
Garst et al[74]	Vinorelbine M-W-F + RT (46 Gy)	36	56%	Esophagitis 19% Dermatitis 8%	20.7 months

[a] AHRT, accelerated hyperfractionated radiotherapy; RT, radiotherapy; CBRT, concomitant boost radiotherapy; HRT, hyperfractionated radiotherapy.
[b] NR, not reported. TID RT three time/day radiotherapy.

therapy; however, the split-course design probably contributed to the lack of benefit. Jeremic et al[69] investigated whether the addition of weekend chemotherapy consisting of carboplatin/etoposide to hyperfractionated radiotherapy and concurrent daily carboplatin/etoposide offers an advantage over the same hyperfractionated radiotherapy/daily carboplatin/etoposide. They treated, in a randomized fashion, 195 patients (98 in group I and 97 in group II) with either hyperfractionated radiation to 69.6 Gy (1.2 Gy twice-daily fractionation) and daily carboplatin and etoposide (50 mg each) during the radiotherapy course (group I) or the same hyperfractionation regimen with daily carboplatin/etoposide (30 mg each) and weekend (Saturdays and Sundays) carboplatin and etoposide (100 mg each) during the radiotherapy course (group II). No differences were found regarding median survival time, 5-year survival rates, and median time to local progression. The 5-year local progression-free survival rates were 28% and 27%, respectively ($p = 0.66$). Weekend chemotherapy did not alter the time to distant metastasis. Increased grade 3 hematologic toxicity was observed in the group receiving the additional weekend chemotherapy ($p = 0.0046$).

Concomitant vinorelbine (20 mg/m^2 on days 1–8), cisplatin (80 mg/m^2 on day 1) every 3 weeks with concurrent hyperfractionated radiotherapy (61 Gy in 5 weeks) in patients with stage III NSCLC demonstrated a 70% response rate, with 78% of the 27 patients experiencing grade 3 leukopenia and neutropenia.[70] Ohashi et al[71] implemented a phase I study of weekly paclitaxel with concurrent hyperfractionated radiotherapy in an effort to determine the MTD of paclitaxel and the DLT of this therapy. Grade 3 lymphocytopenia occurred in 100% of the 15 patients entered into this study, with a response rate of 80%. The design was unusual in that the paclitaxel (starting dose 30 mg/m^2) was delivered every 6 weeks. The DLT was 40 mg/m^2, with 3 of 6 patients developing grade 3 pneumonitis.

The Carolina Lung Cancer Consortium has completed a phase I study of sequential chemoradiotherapy (carboplatin/paclitaxel), noting an MTD of 80 Gy with three-dimensional treatment planning when radiation was delivered in a three times daily fashion.[72] Dose escalation was higher to 86.4 Gy when carboplatin/vinorelbine was employed, with the MTD not being reached. A regimen combining three-times daily radiotherapy to a dose of 57.6 Gy in combination with daily cisplatin determined an MTD of 7.5 mg/m^2/day.[73] The thoracic group at Duke University recently reported their results with concurrent thoracic radiation and vinorelbine delivered three times per week.[74] The median survival was 20.7 months, with a 2-year survival rate of 35% in this group of 36 patients.

Phase I–II trials with 3D conformal radiation alone or with chemotherapy

The incorporation of three-dimensional (3D) radiotherapy techniques has resulted in reduced normal tissue exposure in patients treated for locally advanced NSCLC. Starting with doses ranging from 63 to 84 Gy given in

2.1 Gy fractions, groups from the University of Michigan and the University of South Carolina coordinated a phase I dose-escalation study using 3D conformal radiation in patients with stages I–III or locally recurrent NSCLC.[75] Five groups were created based on the volume of normal lung irradiated, with dose levels chosen based on the estimated risk of radiation pneumonitis. Target volumes included the primary tumor and any nodes 1 cm or larger on computed tomography (CT). Only sites of gross disease were treated. Neoadjuvant cisplatin plus vinorelbine was administered in the latter parts of this study. Of the 104 patients enrolled, 24 had stage I, 4 had stage II, 43 had stage IIIA, 26 had stage IIIB, and 7 had locally recurrent disease. Twenty-five received chemotherapy, and 63 were assessable for escalation. The MTD was only established for the largest group, at 65.1 Gy. Dose levels for the four remaining groups were 102.9, 102.9, 84, and 75.6 Gy. Only two cases of grade 3 radiation pneumonitis occurred. The majority of patients failed distantly, although a significant proportion also failed in the target volume. There were no isolated failures in clinically uninvolved nodal regions.

From 1991 to 1998, 152 patients with stage III NSCLC were treated with 3D conformal radiotherapy at the Memorial Sloan-Kettering Cancer Center.[76] Seventy patients were treated with radiotherapy alone, and 82 received induction chemotherapy with a cisplatin-based regimen prior to receiving radiation. 3D radiation was delivered using CT-based treatment planning (median doses 70.2 Gy with radiation alone and 64.8 Gy with combined therapy). Thirty-nine patients had poor prognostic factors (Karnofsky performance status < 70 or weight loss > 5%), and they were equally distributed between the two groups. The median survivals for the radiation-alone and combined-modality groups were 11.7 months and 18.1 months, respectively ($p = 0.001$). No significant difference was seen in the rates of local control in the radiation-alone and combined-modality groups at 2 years: 35.4% and 43.1%, respectively ($p = 0.1$). Grade 3 or worse non-hematologic toxicity occurred in 20% of the patients receiving radiation alone and in 16% of those receiving chemotherapy and radiation. Overall, there were only four cases of grade 3 or worse esophagitis. Sequential chemoradiotherapy produced a superior survival advantage over 3D conformal radiotherapy alone in stage III NSCLC, despite the higher number of patients with IIIB disease treated on the chemoradiotherapy arm, without a concomitant increase in toxicity.

Graham et al[77] reported the preliminary results of the acute toxicity from RTOG 93-11, a phase I–II dose-escalation study using 3D conformal radiotherapy in patients with inoperable NSCLC. From 1995 to 2001, 163 patients were entered with the goal of establishing the MTD of 3D radiotherapy. Patients were stratified based on the V20 (percentage of total lung volume receiving greater than 20 Gy). The dose range was 70.9–90.3 Gy (the maximum dose allowed was 77.4 Gy for patients with a V20 between 25% and 37%). The MTD at the time of this report had not been reached. Acute toxicity in the form of grade 3/4 pulmonary and esophageal toxicity was modest, with only one grade 3 pneumonitis and esophagitis. Of concern was the observation of 17 grade 3 lung toxicities, with the majority centered in the groups receiving 70–77.4 Gy despite the fact that these patients had V20 < 20 Gy.

Employing 3D conformal radiotherapy leads to the important question as to whether elective nodal irradiation can be omitted in patients with stage III NSCLC. The Rotterdam Oncological Thoracic Study Group entered 54 patients into a phase II study incorporating sequential chemotherapy (two or four cycles of carboplatin/paclitaxel depending on the response to the first two cycles of chemotherapy).[78] Prechemotherapy gross disease (including lymph nodes with a short-axis diameter > 1 cm) was then treated to a dose of 70 Gy using 2 Gy daily fractions with 3D techniques. The recurrence patterns in 47 patients followed for more than 3 months demonstrated no isolated regional recurrences: distant only (8), in-field only (6), in-field and regional (4), and in-field and distant (2). Importantly, no grade 3–5 radiation-induced toxicities were observed, in contrast to the 48% grade 3/4 toxicity seen in RTOG 94-10.

Studies of radiotherapy alone

Many patients with locally advanced NSCLC are not candidates for combined-modality therapy because of comorbid diseases and other reasons. Recently, a retrospective review of 347 patients (1985–1992) with T1 and T2N0M0 tumors treated with radiotherapy alone at the Queensland Radium Institute (QRI) in Australia evaluated whether definitive radiation would provide reasonable outcomes in elderly patients who were unfit for surgery.[79] The median age was 70 years, with the range being 34–90 years. Patients in this group were all treated with standard techniques involving external-beam radiotherapy to a dose of 50 Gy in 20 fractions over 4 weeks. The overall survival rates at 5 years were 22% and 34%, respectively, for patients aged below 70 and for those 70 or older (the median survivals were 22 months for age below 70 and 26 months for age 70 or older). The 5-year disease-free survival rates were 18% for the below-70 group and 30% for the 70 or older group (the median survival was 17 months in both groups). The differences in overall survival and recurrence-free survival between the two age groups approached, but did not reach, statistical significance at the $p < 0.05$ level. Interestingly, the 75- to 79-year group showed better survival than other age groups, with the 5-year overall survival rate for this group being 53%, while the 5-year recurrence-free survival rate was 45%. Thus, elderly patients appear to do just as well with definitive radiotherapy as younger patients, and should be treated similarly.

STAGE IIIB (MALIGNANT PLEURAL EFFUSION)/STAGE IV NSCLC

Since the introduction of platinum-based regimens for NSCLC in the 1980s, evidence has accumulated for the ability of chemotherapy to improve both survival and quality of life in patients with advanced disease in a cost-effective manner. Prior to 1990, standard chemotherapy for patients with unresectable disease and good performance status consisted primarily of cisplatin or carboplatin combined with etoposide, vindesine, vinblastine, ifosfamide, or mitomycin.[80] In a review from 1990 analyzing 27 phase III trials, no one combination of these drugs appeared to have superior efficacy;[81] the same was true of a more recent meta-analysis of 52 trials.[82] Since then, several drugs with substantial ($\geq$ 20%) activity as first-line single agents have been introduced: vinorelbine (a vinca alkaloid microtubule destabilizer), the taxanes paclitaxel and docetaxel (microtubule stabilizers), gemcitabine (a cytarabine-like nucleoside analog), and irinotecan (a topoisomerase I inhibitor).[80] The Eastern Cooperative Oncology Group ECOG 1594 trial compared the utility of some of these newer agents in combination with either carboplatin or cisplatin.[83] Comparable response rates and survival curves suggest that standard doublet chemotherapy has reached a plateau in terms of maximum efficacy. It is important to emphasize, however, that these newer agents with better side-effect profiles have led to modest increases in median survival and 1-year survival rates when compared with standard chemotherapy regimens utilized prior to 1990.

Standard chemotherapy for advanced NSCLC typically consists of a combination of a platinum compound (traditionally considered the most active agents against NSCLC) and one other drug.[84]

While chemotherapy clearly improves survival in these patients, the impact is modest compared with the effectiveness of chemotherapy in other conditions such as Hodgkin lymphoma and germ cell carcinomas. Nevertheless, several phase III studies were conducted and published in 2001 with the hopes of demonstrating better overall survival or perhaps better toxicity profiles.

Three-arm phase III doublets

Four large randomized phase III studies enrolling more than 2600 patients examined various doublet combinations in advanced-stage NSCLC (Table 7.7). The largest trial was the TAX 326 trial, which enrolled 1220 patients and randomized them to docetaxel 75 mg/m^2 on day 1 and cisplatin 75 mg/m^2 on day 1 every 3 weeks versus docetaxel 75 mg/m^2 and carboplatin AUC 6 on day 1 every 3 weeks versus vinorelbine 25 mg/m^2 on days 1, 8, and 15 and cisplatin 100 mg/m^2 on day 1 every 4 weeks.[85–87] After an interim analysis of 592 patients, median survival and 1- and 2-year survival rates favored the docetaxel and cisplatin arm, at 11 months, 47%, and 21%, respectively. Toxicity was comparable across the three arms, although it appears that the cisplatin/vinorelbine arm may have a slightly higher incidence of anemia, nausea, and vomiting. We are awaiting a final analysis in order to determine the statistical significance between these different arms. van Meerbeeck and colleagues[88,89] presented data on their three-arm phase III study with 480 patients. Arm 1 consisted of 159 patients who received cisplatin 80 mg/m^2 on day 1 with paclitaxel 175 mg/m^2 on day 1 every 3 weeks. The 160 patients on arm 2 received

Table 7.7   Three-arm phase III doublets in advanced-stage NSCLC

Authors	No. of patients	Treatment	Overall response rate (%)[a]	Median survival (months)	Survival rate (%)[a] 1-yr	Survival rate (%)[a] 2-yr
Fossella[85] Belani[86] Rodriguez et al[87]	406	Docetaxel 75 mg/m^2 d1 + cisplatin 75 mg/m^2 d1 q3wks *versus*	NR	11	47	21
	406	Docetaxel 75 mg/m^2 d1 + carboplatin AUC 6 d1 q3wks *versus*	NR	9	38	16
	404	Vinorelbine 25 mg/m^2 d1, 8, 15 + cisplatin 100 mg/m^2 d1 q4wks	NR	10	42	14
Smit et al[88] van Meerbeck et al[89]	159	Cisplatin 80 mg/m^2 d1 + paclitaxel 175 mg/m^2 d1 *versus*	31	8	36	NR
	160	Gemcitabine 1250 mg/m^2 d1, 8 + cisplatin 80 mg/m^2 d1 *versus*	36	9	33	NR
	161	Paclitaxel 175 mg/m^2 d1 + gemcitabine 1250 mg/m^2 d1, 8	27	7	27	NR
Alberola et al[90]	410	Cisplatin 100 mg/m^2 d1 + gemcitabine 1250 mg/m^2 d1, 8q3wks *versus*	41	9	NR	NR
		Cisplatin 100 mg/m^2 d1 + gemcitabine 1250 mg/m^2 d1, 8 + vinorelbine 25 mg/m^2 d1, 8 q3wks	40	8	NR	NR

Table 7.7 Continued

Authors	No. of patients	Treatment	Overall response rate (%)[a]	Median survival (months)	Survival rate (%)[a] 1-yr	Survival rate (%)[a] 2-yr
		versus Gemcitabine 1000 mg/m^2 d1, 8 + vinorelbine 30 mg/m^2 d1, 8 + q3wks × 3 then ifosfamide 3 g/m^2 d1 + vinorelbine 30 mg/m^2 d1, 8	24	10	NR	NR
Scagliotti et al[91]	205	Cisplatin 75 mg/m^2 d1 + gemcitabine 1250 mg/m^2 d1, 8 q3wks *versus*	30	10	NR	NR
	201	Carboplatin AUC 6 d1 + paclitaxel 225 mg/m^2 d1 q3wks *versus*	30	10	NR	NR
	201	Cisplatin 100 mg/m^2 d1 + Vinorelbine 25 mg/m^2 qwk × 8 then qwk × 4	32	10	NR	NR

[a] NR, not reported

gemcitabine 1250 mg/m^2 on days 1 and 8 with cisplatin 80 mg/m^2 on day 1 every 3 weeks, while the 161 patients on arm 3 received paclitaxel 175 mg/m^2 on day 1 and gemcitabine 1250 mg/m^2 on days 1 and 8 every 3 weeks. No significant differences were observed in the three arms, with median survivals of 8 months, 9 months, and 7 months, and 1-year survival rates of 36%, 33%, and 27%. Various combinations with gemcitabine were examined by Alberola et al[90] in 410 patients. Patients received gemcitabine 1250 mg/m^2 on days 1 and 8 with cisplatin 100 mg/m^2 on day 1 every 3 weeks in arm 1, while arm 2 consisted of the same regimen with vinorelbine added at 25 mg/m^2 on days 1 and 8. Patients in the third arm were administered gemcitabine 1000 mg/m^2 and vinorelbine 30 mg/m^2 on days 1 and 8 every 3 weeks for three cycles, followed by ifosfamide 3 g/m^2 on day 1 and vinorelbine 30 mg/m^2 on days 1 and 8. While arm 3 had the lowest response rate, at 24%, the median overall survival was the highest, at 10 months (95% confidence interval 5.65–13.2 months). Arms 1 and 2 had equivalent response rates of 41% and 40%, respectively, and median overall survivals of 9 and 8 months, respectively. Compared with historical averages of platinum-based doublets, there does not appear to be an advantage to these different regimens. Scagliotti et al[91] also presented a three-arm phase III doublet trial at the 2001 Meeting of the American Society of Clinical Oncology (ASCO) examining cisplatin and carboplatin in combination with gemcitabine, paclitaxel, or vinorelbine. In this trial, 600 patients were randomized to receive cisplatin 75 mg/m^2 on day 1 with gemcitabine 1250 mg/m^2 on days 1 and 8 or carboplatin AUC 6 on day 1 with paclitaxel 225 mg/m^2 also on day 1 or cisplatin 100 mg/m^2 on day 1 with vinorelbine 25 mg/m^2 every week for 8 weeks. Response rates across all three arms were equivalent, at 30–32%, and median overall survivals were identical, at 10 months. This trial emphasizes that platinum doublets render comparable response and survival rates, as demonstrated in ECOG 1594.[92]

Two-arm phase III doublets

There were several phase III studies that randomized patients to two different arms. The study by Kelly et al[93] examined two platinum arms with cisplatin 100 mg/m^2 on day 1 with vinorelbine 25 mg/m^2 on days 1, 8, 15, and 22 every 4 weeks on arm 1 versus paclitaxel 225 mg/m^2 on day 1 and carboplatin AUC 6 on day 1 given every 3 weeks. This study demonstrated comparable results in both arms, with overall response rates of 28% and 25% and 1-year survivals of 36% and 38% and 2 year survival rates of 16% and 15% respectively. Median overall survival rates were identical at 8 months. The results of these platinum-containing doublets, taken with the results of ECOG 1594 presented at ASCO 2000,[83] reiterate that we have likely reached a plateau of maximum efficacy with platinum-based doublets. While maximum efficacy may be realized with platinum doublets, there is certainly room for improvement with regard to toxicity from platinum-containing regimens. Three other randomized two-arm phase III studies therefore examined the efficacy of a non-platinum arm in comparison with a traditional platinum-containing arm. Kosmidis et al[94]

Table 7.8   Two-arm phase III doublets in advanced-stage NSCLC

Authors	No. of patients	Treatment	Overall response rate (%)	Median survival (months)	Survival rate (%)[a] 1-yr	2-yr
Kelly et al[93]	202	Vinorelbine 25 mg/m^2 d1, 8, 15, 22 + cisplatin 100 mg/m^2 d1 q4wks *versus*	28	8	36	16
	206	Carboplatin AUC 6 d1 + paclitaxel 225 mg/m^2 d1 q3wks	25	8	38	15
Kosmidis et al[94]	249	Paclitaxel 200 mg/m^2 d1 + carboplatin AUC 6 d1 q3wks *versus*	28	10	41	17
	252	Paclitaxel 200 mg/m^2 d1 + gemcitabine 1000 mg/m^2 d1, 8 q3wks	35	10	42	16
Georgoulias et al[95]	205	Docetaxel 100 mg/m^2 d1 + cisplatin 80 mg/m^2 d2 q3wks *versus*	32	10	42	8
	201	Gemcitabine 1100 mg/m^2 d1, 8 + docetaxel 100 mg/m^2 d8 q3wks	30	10	39	8

Table 7.8 Continued

Authors	No. of patients	Treatment	Overall response rate (%)	Median survival (months)	Survival rate (%)[a] 1-yr	2-yr
Sederholm et al[96]	156	Gemcitabine 1250 mg/m² d1, 8 q3wks	12	9	32	5
	135	versus Gemcitabine 1250 mg/m² d1, 8 + carboplatin AUC 5 d1 q3wks	30	11	44	17
Kumitoh et al[97]	151	Cisplatin 80 mg/m² d1 + docetaxel 60 mg/m² d1 q3–4wks	37	11	48	NR
	151	versus Cisplatin 80 mg/m² d1 + vindesine 3 mg/m² d1, 8, 15 q4wks	21	10	43	NR

[a] NR, not reported.

randomized 249 patients to a standard arm consisting of carboplatin AUC 6 and paclitaxel 200 mg/m^2 given on day 1 every 3 weeks and 252 patients to paclitaxel 200 mg/m^2 given on day 1 in combination with gemcitabine 1000 mg/m^2 on days 1 and 8 given every 3 weeks. While an overall response rate of 28% was seen with carboplatin/paclitaxel and a 35% response rate with paclitaxel/gemcitabine, identical survival times were observed, with median overall survivals of 10 months, 1-year survival rates of 41% and 42% and 2 year survival rates of 17% and 16% respectively. Georgoulias et al[95] published the final results of their phase III trial examining docetaxel 100 mg/m^2 given in combination with either cisplatin 80 mg/m^2 or gemcitabine 1100 mg/m^2. Again, comparable response rates of 32% and 30% were witnessed for the docetaxel/cisplatin and gemcitabine/docetaxel arms, respectively. Median overall survivals of 10 months were seen in both arms, with comparable 1-year survival rates of 42% and 39%, respectively, and 2-year survival rates of 8% in both arms. Sederholm[96] examined the need for platinum in combination with gemcitabine in a two-arm phase III study that randomized 156 patients to gemcitabine alone at 1250 mg/m^2 given on days 1 and 8 every 3 weeks versus 135 patients who received the same dose of gemcitabine in combination with carboplatin AUC 5 on day 1 every 3 weeks. This study clearly demonstrates the need for a second agent in front-line therapy for advanced NSCLC, since single-agent gemcitabine resulted in an overall response rate of 12%, with a median overall survival of 9 months and 1- and 2-year survival rates of 32% and 5%. This is compared with carboplatin and gemcitabine, which resulted in an overall response rate of 30%, with a median overall survival of 11 months and 1- and 2-year survival rates of 44% and 17%. While toxicity was less in the gemcitabine-only arm, this was clearly at the cost of efficacy and overall survival. A cisplatin-based two-arm phase III doublet study was conducted by Kunitoh et al[97] in 300 patients randomized to cisplatin 80 mg/m^2 on day 1 with docetaxel 60 mg/m^2 on day 1 or with vindesine 3 mg/m^2 on days 1, 8, and 15. The overall response rates for the two arms were 37% and 21% ($p = 0.002$), with comparable median overall survivals, at 11 and 10 months. The 1-year survival rates were also similar, at 48% and 43%, respectively. These phase III studies demonstrate that the use of two agents in front-line therapy is essential to achieve better response and survival rates. Furthermore, substitution of platinum compounds with one of the newer agents does not appear to be inferior to a traditional platinum-containing doublet and also produces a better toxicity profile.

Phase III triplet regimens

The concept of adding a third agent to standard doublet therapy in order to improve overall response and survival was reflected in four separate publications in 2001. Comella et al[98] compared two different triplet regimens with a control arm of cisplatin 100 mg/m^2 on day 1 with gemcitabine 1000 mg/m^2 given on days 1, 8, and 15 every 4 weeks. The triplet arms consisted of (arm 1)

Table 7.9   Phase III triple chemotherapy studies in advanced-stage NSCLC

Authors	No. of patients	Treatment	Overall response rate (%)	Median survival (months)[a]	Survival rate (%)[a] 1-yr	2-yr
Comella[98]	343	Cisplatin 50 mg/m^2 d1, 8 + gemcitabine 1000 mg/m^2 d1, 8 + vinorelbine 25 mg/m^2 d1, 8 q3wks *versus*	44	12	NR	NR
		Cisplatin 50 mg/m^2 d1, 8 + gemcitabine 1000 mg/m^2 d1, 8 + paclitaxel 125 mg/m^2 d1, 8 q3wks *versus*	48	12	NR	NR
		Cisplatin 100 mg/m^2 d1 + gemcitabine 1000 mg/m^2 d1, 8, 15 q4wks	28	9	NR	NR
Danson et al[99]	124	Mitomycin C 6 mg/m^2 d1 + vinblastine 6 mg/m^2 d1 + cisplatin 100 mg/m^2 d2 q4wks *or* Mitomycin C 6 mg/m^2 d1 + Ifosfamide 3000 mg/m^2 d1 + cisplatin 100 mg/m$_2$ d2 q4wks *versus*	33	NR	NR	NR
	108	Gemcitabine 1000 mg/m^2 d1, 8, 15 + carboplatin AUC 5 d1 q4 wks	32	NR	NR	NR
Camps et al[100]	562	Cisplatin 100 mg/m^2 d1 + gemcitabine 1250 mg/m^2 d1, 8	41	9	NR	NR

Table 7.9 Continued

Authors	No. of patients	Treatment	Overall response rate (%)	Median survival (months)[a]	Survival rate (%)[a] 1-yr	2-yr
		versus Cisplatin 100 mg/m² d1 + gemcitabine 1000 mg/m² d1, 8 + vinorelbine 25 mg/m² d1, 8 q3wks	40	8	NR	NR
		versus Gemcitabine 1000 mg/m² d1, 8 + vinorelbine 30 mg/m² d1, 8 q3wks × 3, then ifosfamide 3 g/m² d1 + vinorelbine 30 mg/m² d1, 8	24	10	NR	NR
Sculier et al[101]	94	Cisplatin 60 mg/m² d1 + carboplatin AUC 3 d1 + ifosfamide 4.5 g/m² d1 q4wks	23	6	23	11
	92	*versus* Cisplatin 60 mg/m² d1 + carboplatin AUC 3 d1 + gemcitabine 1000 mg/m² d1, 8, 15 q4wks	29	8	33	14
	94	*versus* Gemcitabine 1000 mg/m² d1, 8, 15 + ifosfamide 4.5 g/m² d1 q4 wks	25	7	35	17

[a] NR, not reported.

cisplatin 50 mg/m^2, gemcitabine 1000 mg/m^2, and vinorelbine 25 mg/m^2 each given on days 1 and 8 every 3 weeks and (arm 2) cisplatin 50 mg/m^2, gemcitabine 1000 mg/m^2, and paclitaxel 125 mg/m^2 each given on days 1 and 8 every 3 weeks. The overall response rates favored the triplet arms, at 44% and 48%, respectively, compared with a 28% response rate in the gemcitabine/cisplatin standard-chemotherapy arm. This also translated into differences in median overall survival, with the triplet regimens resulting in median survivals of 12 months, compared with 9 months in the control arm. Three other studies evaluating triplet regimens are depicted in Table 7.9. The study by Danson et al[99] evaluated standard mitomycin C /vinblastine/cisplatin or mitomycinc/ifosfamide/cisplatin versus gemcitabine/carboplatin. The response rates were comparable, at around 30%, and toxicity was also comparable between the different arms, although hematologic toxicity appears to be statistically greater in the carboplatin/gemcitabine arm ($p = 0.006$). Gemcitabine regimens were evaluated by Camps et al[100] in a three-arm trial consisting of gemcitabine 1250 mg/m^2 on days 1 and 8 with cisplatin 100 mg/m^2 on day 1 every 3 weeks versus gemcitabine 1000 mg/m^2 on days 1 and 8 with cisplatin 100 mg/m^2 on day 1 and vinorelbine 25 mg/m^2 on days 1 and 8 every 3 weeks versus gemcitabine 1000 mg/m^2 on days 1 and 8 with vinorelbine 30 mg/m^2 on days 1 and 8 every 3 weeks for three cycles followed by ifosfamide 3 g/m^2 on day 1 with vinorelbine 30 mg/m^2 on days 1 and 8. In this study of 562 patients, the response rates were 41%, 40%, and 24% for the three arms, respectively. The median overall survivals were also similar, at 9 months, 8 months, and 10 months, respectively. A fourth study, presented by Sculier et al[101] explored the combination of cisplatin and carboplatin given with either ifosfamide or gemcitabine compared with gemcitabine and ifosfamide. This study demonstrated inferior response rates compared with those cited above, and the median overall survival and 1- and 2-year survival rates were 6–8 months, 23–35%, and 11–17% (Table 7.9). These triplet regimen studies demonstrate that the addition of a third agent may be capable of increasing response rates at the expense of added toxicity, with little benefit to overall survival.

Phase II triplet regimens

Multiple phase II trials involving a three-drug regimen arm were published in 2001.[102–106] Again, the majority of the studies suggest that a third drug does not provide much benefit in terms of overall survival with median survivals ranging from 5.11 months, although initial response rates may be higher ranging from 29%–52% this is at the expense of added toxicity. One study of interest, however, is that by Rosso et al,[102] which randomized 59 patients to a carboplatin/ifosfamide/paclitaxel regimen and 48 patients to a gemcitabine/ifosfamide/vinorelbine regimen. The response rates were 46% and 52% in these two arms, with 1-year survival rates of 43% and 47%. While this is a phase II study, the 1-year survival rates suggests that these regimens may warrant further investigation.

Table 7.10   Phase II triple regimens in advanced-stage NSCLC

Authors	No. of patients	Treatment	Overall response rate (%)	Median survival (months)[a]	Survival rates (%)[a] 1-yr	Survival rates (%)[a] 2-yr
Rosso et al[102]	59	Carboplatin AUC 5 d1 + ifosfamide 3 g/m² d1 + paclitaxel 200 mg/m² d1 q3wks versus	46	NR	43	NR
	48	Gemcitabine 1000 mg/m² d1, 4 + ifosfamide 3 g/m² d1 + vinorelbine 25 mg/m² d1, 4 q3wks	52	NR	47	NR
Souquet et al[103]	259	Vinorelbine 30 mg/m² d1, 8, 15 + cisplatin 80 mg/m² d1 q3wks versus	35	10	38	NR
		Vinorelbine 25 mg/m² d1, 8 + ifosfamide 3 g/m² d1 + cisplatin 75 mg/m² d1 q3wks	36	8	33	NR
Montalar et al[104]	112	Vinorelbine 25 mg/m² d1, 8 + ifosfamide 3 g/m² d1 + cisplatin 80 mg/m² d1 q3wks	50	11	NR	NR
Smith et al[105]	155	Mitomycin C 8 mg/m² d1 courses 1, 2, 4, 6 + vinblastine 6 mg/m² d1 + cisplatin 50 mg/m² d1 q3wks × 6 courses versus	38	6	22	NR
	153	same regimen × 3 courses	31	7	25	NR

Table 7.10   Continued

Authors	No. of patients	Treatment	Overall response rate (%)	Median survival (months)[a]	Survival rates (%)[a] 1-yr	2-yr
Thompson et al[106]	205	Paclitaxel 200 mg/m² d1 + carboplatin AUC 5 d1 + gemcitabine 1000 mg/m² d1, 8	34	10	38	NR
		versus				
		Paclitaxel 200 mg/m² d1 + carboplatin AUC 6 d1 + vinorelbine 20 mg/m² d1, 8, or 15	42	5	32	NR
		versus				
		Paclitaxel 200 mg/m² d1 + gemcitabine 100 mg/m² d1, 8	29	8	40	NR
		versus				
		Gemcitabine 1000 mg/m² d1, 8, 15 + vinorelbine 20 mg/m² d1, 8, 15	29	11	49	NR

[a] NR, not reported.

Two-arm phase II doublets

Three additional randomized studies examined doublet combinations in the phase II setting. Zatlouikal et al[107] compared gemcitabine 1200 mg/m^2 given on days 1 and 8 in combination with either cisplatin 80 mg/m^2 on day 1 or carboplatin AUC 5 on day 1, each given every 3 weeks. While response rates were higher than are traditionally seen, they were comparable at 48% and 47%, respectively. This is certainly encouraging, since the combination of carboplatin and gemcitabine offers a much more favorable side-effect profile with negligible nausea and vomiting and almost no alopecia. This combination is rapidly becoming a predominant first-line doublet given its comparable efficacy and favorable side-effect profile. Another randomized phase II study randomized 51 patients to docetaxel and cisplatin given every 3 weeks and 57 patients to docetaxel and irinotecan also given on a 3-week schedule.[108] The two arms resulted in similar response rates of 37% and 32%, respectively. The median overall survivals were identical, at 11 months, and the 1-year survival rates were 49% and 41%. A study by Grigorescu et al[109] examined cisplatin plus vinblastine versus gemcitabine plus carboplatin. The cisplatin/vinblastine arm proved inferior, with a median overall survival of 8 months and a 1-year survival rate of only 9%. This compares with the carboplatin/gemcitabine arm, which demonstrated a median overall survival of 11 months, with a 1-year survival rate of 20%. These survivals are consistently seen in other studies with carboplatin and gemcitabine. A third study, by Chen et al[110] randomized 90 patients to carboplatin/paclitaxel or paclitaxel/gemcitabine, each administered on a 3-week schedule. Both regimens produced a 40% response rate, with a median overall survival of 10 months in each. Again, a non-platinum doublet appears to provide comparable response rates and survival rates compared with platinum-containing counterparts, and with less toxicity.

Carboplatin-containing phase II doublets

Several phase II studies were published in 2001 examining the efficacy of doublet therapy. Two studies combined docetaxel at doses of 60 or 100 mg/m^2 given on day 1 with carboplatin given at an AUC of 1.9–6.1 or 6 given on 3- or 4-week schedules.[111,112] Response rates were comparable between these two studies, at 37% and 44% (Table 7.12), and median overall survivals were also similar, at 13 months and 12 months. Three other studies explored the efficacy of carboplatin given at an AUC of 6 in combination with paclitaxel at doses ranging from 175 to 225 mg/m^2.[113–115] The response rates were quite variable, ranging from 24% to 46%. The median overall survivals were also variable, ranging between 8 and 15 months, while 1-year survival rates varied from 34% to 50%. Given the number of patients in these three phase II trials, this variability seen with what is considered a standard regimen is not unexpected. Two additional studies administered carboplatin at a fixed dose of 350 mg/m^2 or with an AUC of 4.5 given on day

Table 7.11   Two-arm phase II doublets in advanced-stage NSCLC

Authors	No. of patients	Treatment	Overall response rate (%)	Median survival (months)[a]	Survival rate (%)[a] 1-yr	Survival rate (%)[a] 2-yr
Zatloukal et al[107]	63	Gemcitabine 1200 mg/m^2 d1 8 + cisplatin 80 mg/m^2 d1 q3wks	48	NR	NR	NR
		versus				
		Gemcitabine 1200 mg/m^2 d1, 8 + carboplatin AUC 5 d1 q3wks	47	NR	NR	NR
Satouchi et al[108]	51	Docetaxel 60 mg/m^2 d1 + cisplatin 80 mg/m^2 d1 q3wks	37	11	49	NR
		versus				
	57	Docetaxel 60 mg/m^2 d1 + Irinotecan 60 mg/m^2 d1, 8 q3wks	32	11	41	NR
Grigorescu et al[109]	99	Cisplatin 75 mg/m^2 d1 + Vinblastine 6 mg/m^2 d1, 8 q3wks	15	8	9	NR
		versus				
		Gemcitabine 1000 mg/m^2 d1, 8 + carboplatin 300 mg/m^2 d1 q3wks	27	11	20	NR
Chen et al[110]	90	Paclitaxel 175 mg/m^2 d1 + carboplatin AUC 7 d1 q3wks	40	10	NR	NR
		versus				
		Paclitaxel 175 mg/m^2 d1 + gemcitabine 1000 mg/m^2 d1, 8 q3wks	40	10	NR	NR

[a] NR, not reported.

Table 7.12   Carboplatin-containing phase II doublets in advanced-stage NSCLC

Authors	No. of patients	Treatment	Overall response rate (%)	Median survival (months)[a]	Survival rate (%)[a] 1-yr	2-yr
Bando et al[111]	54	Docetaxel 60 mg/m² d1 + carboplatin AUC 1.9–6.1 d1 q3wks	37	13	56	NR
Zarogoulidis et al[112]	120	Docetaxel 100 mg/m² d1 + carboplatin AUC 6 d1 q4wks	44	12	27	12
Van Kooten et al[113]	136	Carboplatin AUC 6 d1 + paclitaxel 200 mg/m² over 1 h+d1 q3wks	35	15	42	15
Novello et al[114]	60	Carboplatin AUC 6 d1 + paclitaxel 225 mg/m² d1 q3wks	46	12	50	NR
Glorieux et al[115]	130	Carboplatin AUC 6 d1 + paclitaxel 175–200 mg/m² d1 q3wks	24	8	34	NR
Cremonesi et al[116]	53	Carboplatin 350 mg/m² d1 + vinorelbine 25 mg/m² d1, 8 q3wks	26	NR	NR	NR
Bretti et al[117]	83	Carboplatin AUC 4.5 d1 + vinorelbine 25 mg/m² d1, 8 q4wks	31	9	NR	NR

[a] NR, not reported.

1 in combination with vinorelbine 25 mg/m^2 given on days 1 and 8 on either a 3- or a 4-week schedule.[116,117] Response rates were reasonable, at 26% and 31% (Table 7.12). These phase II studies suggest that carboplatin combinations with docetaxel, paclitaxel, or vinorelbine demonstrate comparable response and survival rates.

Cisplatin-containing phase II doublets

Several studies reported the results of cisplatin in combination with gemcitabine, docetaxel, or paclitaxel. A study by Terrioux et al[118] administered gemcitabine 1250 mg/m^2 and cisplatin 50 mg/m^2 given on days 1 and 15 to 56 patients on a 4-week schedule. This resulted in an overall response rate of 34%, with a median overall survival of 10 months. A similarly sized phase II study by Lee et al[119] with 55 patients examined paclitaxel 175 mg/m^2 given on day 1 and cisplatin 75 mg/m^2 on day 2 every 3 weeks. While the overall response rate was a considerable 54%, the median overall survival was only 6 months. A third study, by Ho et al[120] was a larger phase II study with 146 patients, who received cisplatin 75 mg/m^2 and docetaxel 75 mg/m^2 on day 1 every 3 weeks. The overall response rate was 43%, with a significant median overall survival of 14 months. These cisplatin-containing doublets demonstrate that cisplatin continues to offer a role in the first-line treatment of advanced-stage NSCLC.

While the studies cited above clearly argue for a continued benefit of chemotherapy in advanced-stage NSCLC, the side-effect profiles of chemotherapy remain non-trivial. Therefore, much research effort is directed at identifying the least-toxic effective approach to the patient with advanced disease, in order to preserve and maximize quality of life as well as improving survival. To that end, attention has turned to non-platinum doublets and weekly-scheduled chemotherapy regimens.

Non-platinum doublets

There were three phase II doublet studies published in 2001. Two trials examined gemcitabine and paclitaxel, given in combination, however, the dosing and treatment schedules differed in the two studies.[121,122] In the study by Douillard et al,[121] 48 patients were given gemcitabine at a dose of 1000 mg/m^2 on days 1 and 8 in combination with paclitaxel at 200 mg/m^2 on day 1 on a 3 week schedule. The study by Isla et al[122] utilized a higher dose of gemcitabine 2000 mg/m^2 given on days 1 and 15 in combination with paclitaxel at 150 mg/m^2 on days 1 and 15 on a 4 week schedule administered to 89 patients. For these studies, efficacies were comparable, with overall response rates of 36% and 32%, respectively. The median overall survivals were also comparable, at 12 months and 10 months, with 1-year survival rates of 48% and 39%, respectively. Laack et al[123] also examined a non-platinum-containing doublet with gemcitabine at 1000 mg/m^2 on days 1, 8, and 15 given in combination

Table 7.13   Cisplatin-containing phase II doublets in advanced stage NSCLC

Authors	No. of patients	Treatment	Overall response rate (%)	Median survival (months)	Survival rate[a] 1-yr	2-yr
Terrioux et al[118]	56	Gemcitabine 1250 mg/m^2 d1, 15 + cisplatin 50 mg/m^2 d1, 15 q4wks	34	10	NR	NR
Lee et al[119]	55	Paclitaxel 175 mg/m^2 d1 + cisplatin 75 mg/m^2 d2 q3wks	54	6	NR	NR
Ho et al[120]	146	Docetaxel 75 mg/m^2 d1 + cisplatin 75 mg/m^2 d1 q3wks	43	14	NR	NR

[a] NR, not reported.

Table 7.14   Non-platinum doublets in advanced-stage NSCLC

Authors	No. of patients	Treatment	Overall response rate (%)	Median survival (months)	Survival rate (%)[a]	
					1-yr	2-yr
Douillard et al[121]	48	Gemcitabine 1000 mg/m^2 d1, 8 + Paclitaxel 200 mg/m^2 d1 q3wks	36	12	48	NR
Isla et al[122]	89	Gemcitabine 2000 mg/m^2 d1, 15 + Paclitaxel 150 mg/m^2 d1, 15 q4wks	32	10	39	NR
Laack et al[123]	70	Gemcitabine 1000 mg/m^2 d1, 8, 15 + Vinorelbine 30 mg/m^2 d1, 8, 15 q4wks	41	8	34	NR

[a] NR, not reported

with vinorelbine at 30 mg/m^2 also on days 1, 8, and 15 every 4 weeks to 70 patients. The overall response rate was 41%, with a median overall survival of 8 months and a 1-year survival rate of 34%. Each of these regimens proved very tolerable with regard to hematologic and non-hematologic toxicities. Although these studies are all phase II studies, they certainly suggest that non-platinum doublets can be given safely without a compromise in overall response rates and survival. It is hoped that phase III studies with non-platinum-containing combinations will demonstrate non-inferiority to platinum-containing regimens, with greater tolerability, which will likely have a favorable impact on quality of life.

Alternate dosing and weekly chemotherapy regimens

Dosing frequency is another area of interest that has been explored in several studies from 2001. Increasing the frequency of chemotherapy administrations with appropriate dose reductions offers a theoretical reduction in toxicity and perhaps a response benefit as well, since the cancer cells are exposed to chemotherapy more frequently. Belani et al[124,125] explored this concept in a three-arm phase II trial where patients received carboplatin and paclitaxel in various doses and schedules. Carboplatin dosing varied from an AUC of 2 given weekly for 6 out of 8 weeks to an AUC of 6 given once every 4 weeks. Paclitaxel dosing was 150 mg/m^2 reduced to 100 mg/m^2 given weekly for 6 out of 8 weeks and 100 mg/m^2 for the 3 out of 4 weeks schedules. Response rates varied from 18% to 30%, with survival rates favoring the 3-week out of 4 paclitaxel dosing and carboplatin AUC 6 dosed every 4 weeks, with a 1-year survival rate of 48%, compared with 29% and 39% in the other two arms. In another phase II trial, Jagasia et al[126] administered iriniotecan at 65 mg/m^2 weekly for 6 out of 8 weeks concomitantly with cisplatin at 30 mg/m^2, and witnessed a 36% response rate in 50 patients, with a median survival of 12 months and a 1-year survival rate of 46%. While this remains a small phase II study, the concept of weekly chemotherapy is intriguing, with comparable response and survival rates and better toxicity profiles, and awaits the results of phase III studies. One trial examined the role of sequential alternate chemotherapy: Edelman et al[127] randomized 126 patients to receive either carboplatin and gemcitabine followed by paclitaxel or cisplatin and vinorelbine followed by docetaxel. Response rates were comparable, at 21% and 28%, respectively, with identical median overall survivals and 1-year survival rates of 9 months and 32%. Maintenance vinorelbine given at 25 mg/m^2 weekly for 6 months versus observation was explored by Depierre et al[128] in 179 patients, who initially received four cycles of mitomycin C, ifosfamide, and cisplatin. No benefit for maintenance chemotherapy was observed, with a 52% 1-year survival rate seen in the observation arm versus 40% in the maintenance vinorelbine arm. The concept of maintenance chemotherapy remains intuitively attractive, but there is limited data to support its utility.

Table 7.15   Weekly and maintenance regimens in advanced-stage NSCLC

Authors	No. of patients	Treatment	Overall response rate (%)[a]	Median survival (months)	Survival rate (%)[a] 1-yr	2-yr
Belani[124] Belani et al[125]	129	Paclitaxel 100 mg/m^2 d1, 8, 15 + carboplatin AUC 6 d1 q4wks *versus*	30	11	48	NR
	126	Paclitaxel 100 mg/m^2 d1, 8, 15 + carboplatin AUC 2 d1, 8, 15 q4wks *versus*	21	7	29	NR
	123	Paclitaxel 150–100 mg/m^2 d1, 8, 15, 22, 29, 36 + carboplatin AUC 2 d1, 8, 15, 22, 29, 36 q8wks		18	39	NR
Jagasia et al[126]	50	Irinotecan 65 mg/m^2 d1, 8, 15, 22, 29, 36 + cisplatin 30 mg/m^2 d1, 8, 15, 22, 29, 36 q8wks	36	12	46	NR
Edelman et al[127]	126	Carboplatin AUC 5.5 d1 + gemcitabine 1000 mg/m^2 d1, 8 q3wks ×3, then paclitaxel 225 mg/m^2 d1 q3wks ×3 *versus*	21	9	32	NR
		Cisplatin 100 mg/m^2 d1 + vinorelbine 25 mg/m^2 d1, 8q3wks ×3, then docetaxel 75–100 mg/m^2 q3wks ×3	28	9	32	NR
Depierre et al[128]	179	Mitomycin C 6 mg/m^2 d1 + ifosfamide 1.5 g/m^2 d1–3 + cisplatin 30 mg/m^2 d1–3 q4wks ×4, then vinorelbine 25 mg/m^2 qwk × 6 months *versus*	NR	10	40	NR
		Observation	NR	13	52	NR

[a] NR, not reported.

TREATMENT OF ELDERLY AND POOR-PS PATIENTS

A large percentage of NSCLC patients are elderly (age $\geq$ 70 years old), and this is expected to increase. Previously, this subset of patients were denied therapy because age was associated with fragility, rendering patients unable to withstand cytotoxic chemotherapy. The ELVIS trial contradicted this notion by showing a survival benefit for vinorelbine over best supportive care as first line therapy for elderly patients with advanced stage NSCLC.[129] In 2001, two small studies corroborate the role of single-agent chemotherapy in the elderly (Table 7.16). One study evaluated 15 elderly patients treated with vinorelbine and demonstrated a 27% response rate and a 1-year survival rate of 33%, while another study investigated single-agent gemcitabine in 88 patients and reported a response rate of 14%.[130] This second trial continues to accrue patients and includes a randomization to four additional cycles of gemcitabine versus supportive care in non-progressors.[131]

Since doublet therapy is the standard for younger patients, investigators began to evaluate doublet regimens in the elderly (Table 7.16). Encouraging results with pilot trials of vinorelbine plus gemcitabine lead to a phase III trial.[132] The MILES (Multicenter Italian Lung Cancer in the Elderly Study) trial randomized patients 70 years and older to vinorelbine (30 mg/m^2), gemcitabine (1200 mg/m^2), or gemcitabine (1000 mg/m^2) plus vinorelbine (25 mg/m^2). All treatments were given on days 1 and 8 every 21 days. Approximately 700 patients were enrolled into this study. The median age was 74 and the median number of comorbidities was 2. Gemcitabine alone produced less leukopenia and neutropenia as compared with the other two arms, while less thrombocytopenia was noted in the single-agent vinorelbine arm. Non-hematologic toxicities were similar among the groups. Response rates ranged from 17% to 20%. No difference in median survival was observed, with survival times of 37, 28, and 32 weeks, respectively. Thus, the combination regimen did not produce superior results in this trial. Single-agent vinorelbine or gemcitabine remain the standard regimens for the elderly patient.

Meanwhile, other investigators have reviewed their experience with combination chemotherapy for elderly patients. The Southwest Oncology Group (SWOG) reexamined their data from two recently completed phase III trials that administered either cisplatin/vinorelbine or carboplatin/paclitaxel. They reported that older patients represented only 19% of the participants in clinical trials. No statistically significant differences in grade 3–5 toxicities or survival were observed as compared with younger patients.[133] The combination of cisplatin and vinorelbine was not as well tolerated as the carboplatin/paclitaxel regimen in any population. Another retrospective analysis of carboplatin and paclitaxel was conducted from a multi-institutional phase III trial in which chemonaive stage IIIB and IV patients were randomized to receive carboplatin and paclitaxel for four cycles or until progression.[134] Of the 200 patients, 67 (20%) randomized were 70 or older. Again, no differences in toxicities or survival were observed between the age cohorts. This suggests that a platinum-

Table 7.16   Trials in elderly and/or performance status (PS) 2 patients with advanced-stage NSCLC

Authors	No. of patients	Treatment	Response rate (%)	Median survival (months)[a]	1-year survival rate (%)[a]
Lanza et al[130]	15	Vinorelbine 25 mg/m^2 d1, 8, 15 q4wks	27	NR	33
Galli et al[131]	88	Gemcitabine 1500 mg/m^2 d1, 8 q21d	14	NR	NR
MILES[132]	233	Vinorelbine 30 mg/m^2 d1, 8 q21d *versus*	19	37	NR
	233	Gemcitabine 1200 mg/m^2 d1, 8 q21d *versus*	17	28	NR
	232	Vinorelbine 25 mg/m^2 d1, 8 q21d + Gemcitabine 1000 mg/m^2 d1, 8 q21d	20	32	NR
Imperatori et al[135]	31	Vinorelbine 30 mg/m^2 d1, 8, 15 q4wks + Cisplatin 25 mg/m^2 d1, 8, 15 q4wks	32	32	NR
McKay et al[136]	64	Docetaxel 30 mg/m^2 d1, 8, 15 q4wks + Gemcitabine 800 mg/m^2 d1, 8, 15 q4wks	16	30	NR

[a] NR, not reported.

based doublet (particularly with carboplatin) is feasible in the fit elderly. Prospective studies are needed, such as the pilot trial by Imperatori et al,[135] in which weekly cisplatin (25 mg/m^2 on days 1, 8, and 15) and vinorelbine (30 mg/m^2 on days 1, 8, and 15) were given to 31 elderly or poor performance status (PS) patients every 21 days. The overall response rate in the 22 evaluable patients was 47% (3 complete and 7 partial responses), while it was 33% for all 31 patients. The median survival time was 32 weeks. The most frequent toxicity was grade 3 and 4 neutropenia, which developed in 32% and 13% of patients, respectively. All other toxicities were rare. Finally, McKay et al[136] from the Minnie Pearl Cancer Center conducted a phase II trial of a non-platinum doublet (docetaxel and gemcitabine) in elderly or poor-risk patients. Patients received docetaxel 30 mg/m^2 with gemcitabine 800 mg/m^2, weekly for 3 or 4 weeks. Sixty-four elderly patients with an average age of 71 were enrolled into the trial. Twenty-eight percent of the patients had a PS of 2. An objective response rate of 16% was achieved, with a median survival of 30 weeks. The regimen was well tolerated, with grade 3 or 4 leukopenia, thrombocytopenia, and asthenia developing in 11%, 11%, and 14% of patients, respectively.

OTHER MEDICAL TREATMENTS (INCLUDING BIOLOGIC THERAPY)

A number of trials in 2001 attempted to incorporate biologic agents into NSCLC therapy, but the majority of these studies were phase I or II studies with several having less than 50 patients per study. These agents and their associated studies are presented in Table 7.17. From these data, it does appear that trastuzumab has a fairly limited role to play in the treatment of advanced-stage NSCLC.[137–139] Its combination with traditional chemotherapy regimens does not appear to result in higher response rates or overall survival. However, a drug such as trastuzumab may still hold promise in a select group of patients who overexpress the HER2/neu (c-ErbB-2) receptor to a high degree. Future studies would need to limit enrollment to those patients who have high expression of HER2/neu in the hope of generating beneficial response rates and overall survivals.

Another molecularly targeted agent worthy of mention based on early data is presented in the study by Yuen et al[140] which gave 48 patients carboplatin AUC 6 and paclitaxel 175 mg/m^2 on day 4 in combination with the protein kinase C α (PKCα) antisense drug ISIS-3521. This regimen resulted in an overall response rate of 42%, with a median overall survival of 16 months and an impressive 1-year survival rate of 75%. We eagerly await the results of two phase III studies examining this compound with carboplatin and paclitaxel as well as with cisplatin and gemcitabine.

Trials incorporating the molecularly targeted agents prinomastat and RhuMab-VEGF (a recombinant human monoclinical antibody directed against vascular endothelial growth factor) were also reported on in 2001. While prinomastat does not appear to add significantly to overall response rates or survivals,[141] data from Johnson et al[142] from Vanderbilt University suggest an improvement in overall response rate, median survival, and 1-year survival rate with RhuMab-VEGF when given in combination with carboplatin and paclitaxel. The primary end of this trials, time to progression was statistically superior for the 15 mg/kg arm when compared to the control ($p = 0.02$).

While the results of phase III studies incorporating molecularly targeted agents into traditional chemotherapy regimens remain premature, there is a cautious optimism, which will likely be reflected in future study designs for the treatment of advanced-stage NSCLC.

SECOND-LINE THERAPY IN NSCLC

Recent data have demonstrated the benefit of chemotherapy in the second-line setting. Two phase III studies have shown that single-agent docetaxel provides not only a quality-of-life benefit, but also an improvement in overall survival.[143] Several studies were published this past year examining the role of single-agent therapy as well as doublet therapy in the setting of relapsed or recurrent NSCLC.

Single-agent gemcitabine was examined by van Putten et al[144] in a phase II study with 80 patients, who were given gemcitabine at a dose of 1000 mg/m^2 on a 4-week schedule on days 1, 8, and 15. This schedule resulted in an overall response rate of 13%, which is comparable to the 7% response rate seen with single-agent docetaxel. The median overall survival was 6 months and the 1-year survival rate was 22%. Gemcitabine was also examined in combination with docetaxel in two phase II studies. In the study by Kosmas et al,[145] gemcitabine was administered at 1000 mg/m^2 on days 1, 8, and 15, with docetaxel at 100 mg/m^2 on day 1, on a 4-week schedule. In 41 evaluable patients, a response rate of 33% and a median survival of 9 months were seen. At 1 year, 28% of patients were alive. A comparable study by Spiridonidis et al[146] examined a similar regimen of gemcitabine at 800 mg/m^2 on days 1, 8, and 15, with docetaxel at 100 mg/m^2 on day 1, on a 4-week schedule. This yielded a comparable response rate of 33%, with a median overall survival of 8 months.

Agelaki et al[147] explored two different doublet regimens in two simultaneous phase II studies. One doublet regimen gave vinorelbine 25 mg/m^2 on days 1 and 8, with ifosfamide 1.6 g/m^2 on days 8, 9, and 10, every 4 weeks, to 26 patients. This led to a low response rate of 3% with a median overall survival of 6 months and a 1-year survival rate of 19%. In a second phase II study, 29 patients received carboplatin 300 mg/m^2 on day 1 in combination with vinorelbine 30 mg/m^2 given on days 1 and 8 every 4 weeks. This led to a response rate of 16% with a median overall survival of 9 months and a 1-year survival rate of 38%. These doublet combinations proved to be tolerable regimens, suggesting that such doublet combinations warrant further investigation in phase III studies.

Table 7.17   Molecularly targeted agents in NSCLC

Authors	No. of patients	Treatment	Overall response rate (%)	Median survival (months)[a]	Survival rate (%)[a] 1-yr	Survival rate (%)[a] 2-yr
Zinner et al[137]	12	Cisplatin 75 mg/m² d1 + Gemcitabine 1250 mg/m² d1, 8 q3wks × 6, then Trastuzumab 2 mg/kg weekly	50	NR	NR	NR
Krug et al[138]	39	Docetaxel 36 mg/m² qwk × 6 + Trastuzumab 2 mg/kg qwk q2mos versus Paclitaxel 90 mg/m² qwk × 6 + Trastuzumab 2 mg/kg qwk q2mos	26	NR	NR	NR
			26	NR	NR	NR
Langer et al[139]	51	Carboplatin AUC 6 d1 + Paclitaxel 225 mg/m² d1 + Trastuzumab 2 mg/m² qwk q3wks	18	9.8	NR	NR
Yuen et al[140]	48	Carboplatin AUC 6 d4 + Paclitaxel 175 mg/m² d4 + ISIS-3521 2 mg/kg/d d1–14 q3wks	42	16	75%	NR
Smylie et al[141]	198	Paclitaxel 200 mg/m² d1 q3wks Carboplatin AUC 6 d1 + placebo	21	10	29%	NR
	84	'P + C' + prinomastat 5 mg p.o. bid	27	9	30%	NR
	197	'P + C' + prinomastat 10 mg p.o. bid	19	9	35%	NR
	198	'P + C' + prinomastat 15 mg p.o. bid	18	9	40%	NR

[a]P + C = Paclitaxel + carboplatin.

Table 7.17 Continued

Authors	No. of patients	Treatment	Overall response rate (%)	Median survival (months)[a]	Survival rate (%)[a] 1-yr	Survival rate (%)[a] 2-yr
Johnson et al[142]	25	Carboplatin AUC 6 d1 + paclitaxel 200 mg/m² d1 q3wks	12	12	NR	NR
		versus				
	22	'P + C' + RhuMab-VEGF 7.5 mg/kg	32	14	NR	NR
		versus				
	31	'P + C' + RhuMab-VEGF 15.0 mg/kg	32	18	NR	NR

[a] NR, not reported.
'P + C' = Paclitaxel + carboplatin.

Table 7.18 Second-line treatment for NSCLC

Authors	No. of patients	Treatment	Response rate (%)	Median survival (months)	1-year survival rate (%)[a]
van Putten et al[144]	80	Gemcitabine 1000 mg/m^2, d1, 8, 15 q28d	13	6	22%
Kosmas et al[145]	41	Gemcitabine 1000 mg/m^2, d1, 8, 15 + Docetaxel 100 mg/m^2, d1 q28d	33	9	28%
Spiridonidis et al[146]	40	Gemcitabine 800 mg/m^2 d1, 8, 15 + Docetaxel 100 mg/m^2, d1 q4wks	33	8	NR
Agelaki et al[147]	26	Vinorelbine 25 mg/m^2 d1, 8 + Ifosfamide 1.6 g/m^2 d8–10 q4wks	3	6	19%
Agelaki et al[147]	29	Vinorelbine 30 mg/m^2 d1, 8 + Carboplatin 300 mg/m^2 d1 q4wks	16	9	38%

[a] NR, not reported.

REFERENCES

1. Naruke T, Tsuchiya R, Kondo H et al. Prognosis and survival after resection for bronchogenic carcinoma based on the 1997 TNM-staging classification: the Japanese experience. *Ann Thorac Surg* 2001; **71**: 1759–64.

2. Solaini L, Prusciano F, Bagioni P et al. Video-assisted thoracic surgery major pulmonary resections: present experience. *Eur J Cardio-Thorac Surg* 2001; **20**: 437–42.

3. Nomori H, Horio H, Naruke T et al. What is the advantage of thoracoscopic lobectomy over a limited thoracotomy procedure for lung cancer surgery? *Ann Thorac Surg* 2001; **72**: 879–84.

4. Koizumi K, Haraguchi S, Hirata T et al. Video-assisted lobectomy in elderly lung cancer patients. *Jpn J Thorac Cardiovasc Surg* 2002; **50**: 15–22.

5. Okada M, Yoshikawa K, Hatta T et al. Is segmentectomy with lymph node assessment an alternative to lobectomy for non-small cell lung cancer of 2 cm or smaller? *Ann Thorac Surg* 2001; **71**: 956–60.

6. Miller DL, Rowland CM, Deschamps C et al. Surgical treatment of non-small cell lung cancer 1 cm or less in diameter. *Ann Thorac Surg* 2002; **73**: 1545–51.

7. Ohta Y, Oda M, Wu J et al. Can tumor size be a guide for limited surgical intervention in patients with peripheral non-small cell lung cancer? Assessment from the point of view of nodal micrometastasis. *J Thorac Cardiovasc Surg* 2001; **122**: 900–6.

8. Watanabe S, Oda M, Go T et al. Should mediastinal nodal dissection be routinely undertaken in patients with peripheral small-sized (2 cm or less) lung cancer? Retrospective analysis of 225 patients. *Eur J Cardio-Thoracic Surg* 2001; **20**: 1007–11.

9. Wu Y, Wang S, Huang Z. Extent of lymphadenectomy in stage I–IIIA non-small cell lung cancer: a randomized clinical trial. *Chung-Hua Chung Liu Tsa Chih [Chin J Oncol]* 2001; **23**: 43–5.

10. Sagawa M, Sato M, Sakurada A et al. A prospective trial of systematic nodal dissection for lung cancer by video-assisted thoracic surgery: Can it be perfect? *Ann Thorac Surg* 2002; **73**: 900–4.

11. Elia S, Griffo S, Gentile M et al. Surgical treatment of lung cancer invading chest wall: a retrospective analysis of 110 patients. *Eur J Cardio-Thoracic Surg* 2001; **20**: 356–60.

12. Magdeleinat P, Alifano M, Benbrahem C et al. Surgical treatment of lung cancer invading the chest wall: results and progrnostic actors. *Ann Thorac Surg* 2001; **71**: 1094–9.

13. Facciolo F, Cardillo G, Lopergolo M et al. Chest wall invasion in non-small cell lung carcinoma: a rationale for en bloc resection. *J Thorac Cardiovasc Surg* 2001; **121**: 649–56.

14. McGarry RC, Song G, des Rosiers P et al. Observation-only management of early stage, medically inoperable lung cancer: poor outcome. *Chest* 2002; **121**: 1155–8.

15. Uematsu M, Shioda A, Suda A et al. Computed tomography-guided frameless stereotactic radiotherapy for stage I non-small cell lung cancer: a 5-year experience. *Int J Radiat Oncol Biol Phys* 2001; **51**: 666–70.

16. Gilson B, Glassman J, Bockowski D et al. Body stereotactic radiosurgery (BSR) for primary extracranial tumors. *Proc ASCO* 2001; **20**: 325a.

17. Kang S, Luo R, Liao W et al. Effects of radiofrequency ablation on lung cancer. *Proc ASCO* 2001; **20**: 336a.

18. Rosell R, Felip E, Maestre J et al. The role of chemotherapy in early

non-small-cell lung cancer management. *Lung Cancer* 2001; **34:** (Suppl 3): S63–74.

19. Pisters KMW. Adjuvant and neoadjuvant therapy for early stage non-small cell lung cancer. *Semin Oncol* 2001; **28:** 23–28.

20. Movsas B. Role of adjuvant therapy in resected stage II/IIIA non-small-cell lung cancer. *Oncology* 2001; **15:** 1549–58.

21. Trodella L, Granone P, Valente S et al. Adjuvant radiotherapy in non-small cell lung cancer with pathological stage I: definitive results of a phase III randomized trial. *Radiother Oncol* 2002; **62:** 11–19.

22. Xu G, Rong T, Lin P. Adjuvant chemotherapy following radical surgery for non-small-cell lung cancer: a randomized study on 70 patients. *Chin Med J* 2000; **113:** 617–20.

23. Mineo TC, Ambrogi V, Corsaro V et al. Postoperative adjuvant therapy for stage IB non-small-cell lung cancer. *Eur J Cardio-Thorac Surg* 2001; **20:** 378–84.

24. Kato H, Konaka C, Tsuboi M et al. Randomized Phase III study comparing ubenimex (Bestatin®) versus placebo as postoperative adjuvant treatment in patients with stage I squamous cell lung cancer. *Proc ASCO* 2001; **20:** 307a.

25. Sakamoto J, Teramukai S, Watanabe Y et al. Meta-analysis of adjuvant immunochemotherapy using OK-432 in patients with resected non-small-cell lung cancer. *J Immunother* 2001; **24:** 250–6.

26. Landareneau RL, Szwerc MF, Hen AF et al. Intraoperative brachytherapy with ^{125}I following resection for patients with stage I NSCLC. *Proc ASCO* 2001; **20:** 310a.

27. Depierre A, Westeel V. Overview of the role of neoadjuvant chemotherapy for early stage non-small cell lung cancer. *Semin Oncol* 2001; **28:** 29–36.

28. Marks R, Streitz J, Deschamps C et al. Response rate and toxicity of pre-operative paclitaxel and carboplatin in patients with resectable non-small cell lung cancer. *Proc ASCO* 2001; **20:** 340a.

29. Breton JP, Westeel V, Milleron B et al. Postoperative morbidity and mortality after neoadjuvant chemotherapy (NCT) for non small cell lung cancer (NSCLC) in the French phase III trial. *Proc ASCO* 2001; **20:** 311a.

30. Martin J, Ginsberg RJ, Abolhoda A et al. Morbidity and mortality after neoadjuvant therapy for lung cancer: the risks of right pneumonectomy. *Ann Thorac Surg* 2001; **72:** 1149–54.

31. Roberts JR, Eustis C, Devore R et al. Induction chemotherapy increases perioperative complications in patients undergoing resection for non-small cell lung cancer. *Ann Thorac Surg* 2001; **72:** 885–8.

32. Novoa N, Varela G, Jimenez MF. Morbidity after surgery for non-small cell lung carcinoma is not related to neoadjuvant chemotherapy. *Eur J Cardio-Thorac Surg* 2001; **20:** 700–4.

33. Ichinose Y, Kato H, Koike T et al. Overall survival and local recurrence of 406 completely resected stage IIIa–N2 non-small cell lung cancer patients: questionnaire survey of the Japan Clinical Oncology Group to plan for clinical trials. *Lung Cancer* 2001; **34:** 29–36.

34. Bueno R, Richards WG, Swanson SJ. Nodal stage after induction therapy for stage IIIA lung cancer determines patient survival. *Ann Thorac Surg* 2000; **70:** 1826–31.

35. Albain KS, Crowley JJ, Turrisi AT 3rd et al. Concurrent cisplatin, etoposide, and chest radiotherapy in pathologic stage IIIB non-small-cell lung cancer: a Southwest Oncology Group phase II study, SWOG 9019. *J Clin Oncol* 2002; **20:** 3454–60.

36. Ichinose Y, Tada H, Koike T et al. A randomized phase III trial of postoperative adjuvant chemotherapy in patients with completely resected stage IIIa–N2 non-small cell lung cancer: Japan Clinical Oncology Group (JCOG 9304) trial. *Proc ASCO* 2001; **20**: 311a.

37. Wolf M, Muller H, Seifart U et al. Randomized Phase III trial of adjuvant radiotherapy versus adjuvant chemotherapy followed by radiotherapy in patients with N2 positive non small cell lung cancer. *Proc ASCO Oncol* 2001; **20**: 311a.

38. Greco FA, Burris HA 3rd, Gray JR et al. Paclitaxel and carboplatin adjuvant therapy alone or with radiotherapy for resected nonsmall cell lung carcinoma: a feasibility study of the Minnie Pearl Cancer Research Network. *Cancer* 2001; **92**: 2142–7.

39. Eberhardt W, Bildat S, Korfee S et al. Preoperative treatment strategies in stage III non-small cell lung cancer. *Lung Cancer* 2001; **33** (Suppl 1): S51–9.

40. Spasova I, Petera J, Hytych V. The role of neoadjuvant chemotherapy in marginally resectable or unresectable stage III non-small cell lung cancer. *Neoplasma* 2002; **49**: 189–96.

41. Santo A, Pedersini R, Pasini F et al. A phase II study of induction chemotherapy with gemcitabine (G) and cisplatin (P) in locally advanced non-small cell lung cancer: interim analysis. *Lung Cancer* 2001; **34**(Suppl 4): S15–20.

42. Yang CH, Tsai CM, Wang LS et al. Gemcitabine and cisplatin in a multimodality treatment for local advanced non-small cell lung cancer. *Br J Cancer* 2002; **86**: 190–5.

43. Voltolini L, Luzzi L, Ghiribelli C et al. Results of induction chemotherapy followed by surgical resection in patients with stage IIIA (N2) non-small cell lung cancer: the importance of the nodal downstaging after chemotherapy. *Eur J Cardio-Thoracic Surg* 2001; **20**: 1106–12.

44. Weitberg AB, Liu L, Yashar J et al. Twelve-year follow-up of trimodality therapy for stage IIIA non-small cell lung cancer. *J Exp Clin Cancer Res* 2001; **20**: 335–40.

45. Wright CD, Menard MT, Wain JC et al. Induction chemoradiation compared with induction radiation for lung cancer involving the superior sulcus. *Ann Thorac Surg* 2002; **73**: 1541–4.

46. Raefsky E, Hainsworth J, Burris H et al. Weekly paclitaxel and carboplatin with radiotherapy as preoperative therapy for patients with stage IIB and III non-small cell lung cancer: a Minnie Pearl Cancer Research Network Trial. *Proc ASCO* 2001; **20**: 329a.

47. Ahn YC, Park K, Kim DY et al. Preoperative concurrent chemoradiotherapy for stage IIIA non-small cell lung cancer. *Acta Oncol* 2001; **40**: 588–92.

48. Andre F, Grunenwald D, Pujol JL et al. Patterns of relapse of N2 nonsmall-cell lung carcinoma patients treated with preoperative chemotherapy: Should prophylactic cranial irradiation be reconsidered? *Cancer* 2001; **91**: 2394–400.

49. Anon. Chemotherapy in non-small cell lung cancer: a meta-analysis using updated data on individual patients from 52 randomised clinical trials. Non-Small Cell Lung Cancer Collaborative Group. *BMJ* 1995; **311**: 1411–22.

50. Pritchard RS, Anthony SP. Chemotherapy plus radiotherapy compared with radiotherapy alone in the treatment of locally advanced, unresectable, non-small cell lung cancer: a meta-analysis. *Ann Intern Med* 1996; **125**: 723–9.

51. Furuse K, Fukuoka M, Kawahara M et al. Phase III study of concurrent versus sequential thoracic radiother-

apy in combination with mitomycin, vindesine, and cisplatin in resectable stage III non-small cell lung cancer. *J Clin Oncol* 1999; **17**: 2692–9.

52. Curran WJ Jr, Scott C, Langer C et al. Phase III comparison of sequential vs concurrent chemoradiation for patients with unresectable stage III non-small cell lung cancer (NSCLC): initial report of Radiation Therapy Oncology Group (RTOG-9410). *Proc ASCO* 2000; **19**: 484a.

53. Curran WJ, et al, Initial report of locally advanced multimodality protocol (LAMP): ACR 427: a randomized 3-arm phase II study of pacflitaxel (T), carboplatin (C) and thoracic radiation (TRT) for patients with stage III NSCLC. *Proc ASCO* 2001; **20**: 312a.

54. Vokes EE. Induction chemotherapy followed by concomitant chemoradiotherapy for non-small-cell lung cancer. *Oncologist* 2001; **6**(Suppl 1): 25–7.

55. Langer CJ, Hsu C, Curran W et al. Do elderly patients (pts) with locally advanced non-small cell lung cancer (NSCLC) benefit from combined modality therapy? A secondary analysis of RTOG 94–10. *Proc ASTRO* 2001; **51** (Suppl 1): 20.

56. Komaki R, Lee JS, Kaplan P. Randomized phase III study of amifostine in patients treated with chemoradiation for inoperable stage II–III non-small cell lung cancer (NSCLC). *Proc ASTRO* 2001; **51**(Suppl 1): 19.

57. Guichard N, Dohollu O, Dahan L et al. Phase II trial of weekly paclitaxel, carboplatin and concurrent radiation therapy for locally advanced non-small cell lung cancer (NSCLC). *Proc ASCO* 2001; **20**: 257b.

58. Sirzen F, Lamberg K, Mrazek E et al. Phase II study in weekly paclitaxel and carboplatin and concurrent thoracic radiation therapy (TRT) for locally advanced non-small cell lung cancer (NSCLC). *Proc ASCO* 2001; **20**: 254b.

59. Rosenman JG, Halle JS, Socinski MA et al. High-dose conformal radiotherapy of stage IIIA/IIIB non-small cell lung cancer: technical issues and results of a phase I/II trial. *Int J Radiat Oncol Biol Phys* 2002; **54**: 348–56.

60. Lau D, Leigh B, Gandara D et al. Twice-weekly paclitaxel and weekly carboplatin with concurrent thoracic radiation followed by carboplatin/paclitaxel consolidation for stage III non-small-cell lung cancer: a California Cancer Consortium phase II trial. *J Clin Oncol* 2001; **19**: 442–7.

61. George CM, Mauer DJ, Haraf D et al. Induction chemotherapy (CT) and concomitant chemoradiotherapy (CRT) with carboplatin (C), paclitaxel (P) and irinotecan (I) for unresectable stage III non-small cell lung cancer (NSCLC): a phase I study. *Proc ASCO* 2001; **20**: 242b.

62. Somer R, Langer C, Movsas B et al. Phase I study of irinotecan (CPT-11), cisplatin (cDDP) and radical thoracic radiation (TRT) in the treatment of locally advanced non-small cell lung cancer (NSCLC). *Proc ASCO* 2001; **20**: 258b.

63. Sakai H, Yoneda Y, Noguchi Y et al. A phase I/II study of bi-weekly docetaxel (DOC) and carboplatin (CBDCA) with concurrent thoracic radiation therapy (TRT) followed by consolidation chemotherapy with DOC/CBDCA for stage III unresectable non-small cell lung cancer (NSCLC). *Proc ASCO* 2001; **20**: 238b.

64. Choy H, DeVore RF, Hande KR et al. Phase I trial of outpatient weekly docetaxel, carboplatin and concurrent thoracic radiation therapy for stage III unresectable non-small-cell lung cancer: a Vanderbilt Cancer Center Affiliate Network (VCCAN) trial. *Lung Cancer* 2001; **34**: 441–9.

65. Carabantes F, Cobo M, Gil S et al. Phase II study of neoadjuvant and concurrent chemo-radiotherapy with cisplatin (CDDP) and vinorelbine (VRL) in advanced stage (stage III-B) non-small cell lung cancer (NSCLC). *Proc ASCO* 2001; 20: 2830.

66. Skarin AT, Sugerbaker D, Berman D et al. Phase I study of carboplatin (CAR) and docetaxel (DOC) followed by weekly CAR/DOC with concurrent radiotherapy (CT/RT) in stage III NSCLC. *Proc ASCO* 2001; 20: 277b.

67. Blackstock WA, Lesser GL, Fletcher-Steede J et al. Phase I study of twice-weekly gemcitabine and concurrent thoracic radiation for patients with locally advanced non-small cell lung cancer. *Int J Radiat Oncol Biol Phys* 2001; 51: 1281–9.

68. Schild SE, Stella PJ, Geyer SM et al. Phase III trial of chemotherapy plus once daily or twice daily radiotherapy in stage III non-small cell lung cancer. *In J Radiat Oncol Biol Phys* 2002; 54: 370–8.

69. Jeremic B, Shibamoto Y, Acimovic L et al. Hyperfractionated radiation therapy and concurrent low-dose, daily carboplatin/etoposide with or without weekend carboplatin/etoposide chemotherapy in stage III non-small-cell lung cancer: a randomized trial. *Int J Radiat Oncol Biol Phys* 2001; 50: 19–25.

70. Kisohara A, Simuzu T, Uehara N et al. Phase II study of navelbine (NVB)–cisplatin (CDDP) combination chemotherapy with concurrent radiation in non small cell lung cancer. *Proc ASCO* 2001; 20: 240b.

71. Ohashi N, Arita K, Daido K et al. Phase I study of weekly paclitaxel with concurrent hyperfractionated radiation therapy for advanced non-small cell lung cancer. *Proc ASCO* 2001; 20: 2810.

72. Marks LB, Hurst J, Socinski MA. The maximally tolerated dose of accelerated hyperfractionated conformal radiation therapy (RT) following carboplatin/paclitaxel or carboplatin/navelbine (CN) for unresectable non-small cell lung cancer: a phase I dose escalation study from the Carolina Conformal Therapy Consortium. *Proc ASCO* 2001; 20: 330a.

73. Schild SE, Wong WW, Halyard MY. TID radiotherapy (RT) and escalating doses of daily cisplatin (CDDP) for stage III non-small cell lung cancer (NSCLC): toxicity, tumor response and survival. *Proc ASCO* 2001; 20: 331a.

74. Garst J, Shafman T, Campagna L. A Phase II study of concurrent multidose vinorelbine with definitive radiation therapy for inoperable stage III non-small cell lung cancer (NSCLC). *Proc ASCO* 2001; 20: 343a.

75. Hayman JA, Martel MK, Ten Haken RK et al. Dose escalation in non-small-cell lung cancer using three-dimensional conformal radiation therapy: update of a phase I trial. *J Clin Oncol* 2001; 19: 127–36.

76. Sim S, Rosenzweig KE, Schindelheim R et al. Induction chemotherapy plus three-dimensional conformal radiation therapy in the definitive treatment of locally advanced non-small-cell lung cancer. *Int J Radiat Oncol Biol Phys* 2001; 51: 660–5.

77. Graham MV, Winter K, Purdy JA et al. Preliminary results of a radiation therapy oncology group trial (RTOG 9311), a dose escalation study using 3D conformal radiation therapy in patients with inoperable nonsmall cell lung cancer. *Proc ASTRO* 2001; 51(Suppl 1): 19.

78. Senan S, Burgers JA, Samson MJ et al. Can elective nodal irradiation be omitted in stage III non-small cell lung cancer? An analysis of recurrences after sequential chemotherapy and 'involved-field' radiotherapy to 70 Gy. *Proc ASTRO* 2001; 51(Suppl 1): 21.

79. Gauden SJ, Tripcony L. The curative treatment by radiation therapy

alone of stage I non-small cell lung cancer in a geriatric population. *Lung Cancer* 2001; **32**: 71–9.

80. Bunn PAJ, Kelly K. New treatment agents for advanced small cell and non-small cell lung cancer. *Semin Oncol* 1995; **22**: 53–63.

81. Slinter TA. Chemotherapy in advanced non-small cell lung cancer. *Eur J Cancer* 1990; **26**: 1093–9.

82. Non-small cell Lung Cancer Collaborative Group. Chemotherapy in non-small cell lung cancer: a meta-analysis using updated data on individual patients from 52 randomised clinical trials. *BMJ* 1995; **311**: 899–909.

83. Schiller JH, Harrington D, Sandler A et al. A randomized phase III trial of four chemotherapy regimens in advanced non-small cell lung cancer. *Proc ASCO* 2000; **19**: 1a.

84. Clinical practice guidelines for the treatment of unresectable non-small cell lung cancer. Adopted on May 16, 1997 by the American Society of Clinical Oncology. *J Clin Oncol* 1997; **15**: 2996–3018.

85. Fossella F. Docetaxel + cisplatin (DC) and docetaxel + carboplatin (DCb) vs vinorelbine + cisplatin (VC) in chemotherapy-naïve patients with advanced and metastatic non-small cell lung cancer (NSCLC): results of a multi-center, randomized phase III study. *Eur J Cancer* 2001; **37**: 154.

86. Belani C. Phase III randomized trial of docetaxel in combination with cisplatin or carboplatin or vinorelbine plus cisplatin in advanced non-small cell lung cancer: interim analysis. *Semin Oncol* 2001; **28**: 10–14.

87. Rodriguez J, Pawel J, Pluzanska A et al. A multicenter, randomized phase III study of docetaxel + cisplatin and docetaxel + carboplatin vs vinorelbine + cisplatin in chemotherapy-naive patients with advanced and metastatic non-small

cell lung cancer. *Proc ASCO* 2001; **20**: 314a.

88. Smit E, van Meerbeeck J, Lianes P et al. An EORTC randomized phase III trial of three chemotherapy regimens in advanced non-small cell lung cancer. *Eur J Cancer* 2001; **37**: 154.

89. van Meerbeeck JP, Smit EF, Lianes P et al. A EORTC randomized phase III trial of three chemotherapy regimens in advanced non-small cell lung cancer. *Proc ASCO* 2001; **20**: 308a.

90. Alberola VCM, Provencia M, Isla D et al. Cisplatin/gemcitabine vs cisplatin/gemcitabine/vinorelbine vs sequential doublets of gemcitabine/vinorelbine followed by ifosfamide/vinorelbine in advanced non-small cell lung cancer: results of a Spanish Lung Cancer Group phase III trial. *Proc ASCO* 2001; **20**: 308a.

91. Scagliotti GV, De Marinis F, Rinaldi M et al. Phase III randomized trial comparing three platinum based doublets in advanced non-small cell lung cancer. *Proc ASCO* 2001; **20**: 308a.

92. Schiller JH, Harrington D, Belani CP et al. Comparison of four chemotherapy regimens for advanced non-small-cell-lung-cancer. *N Engl J Med* 2002; **346**: 92–8.

93. Kelly K, Crowley J, Bunn PA Jr et al. Randomized phase III trial of paclitaxel plus carboplatin versus vinorelbine plus cisplatin in the treatment of patients with advanced non-small-cell lung cancer: a Southwest Oncology Group trial. *J Clin Oncol* 2001; **19**: 3210–18.

94. Kosmidis P, Bacoyiannis C, Mylonakis N et al. Paclitaxel plus carboplatin versus paclitaxel plus gemcitabine in advanced NSCLC. Final results of a randomized phase III study. *Eur J Cancer* 2001; **37**: 28.

95. Georgoulias V, Papadakis E, Alexopoulos A et al. Platinum-

based and non-platinum-based chemotherapy in advanced non-small-cell lung cancer: a randomised multicentre trial. *Lancet* 2001; **37**: 1478–84.

96. Sederholm C. A phase III study in advanced non-small cell lung cancer comparing gemcitabine with gemcitabine in combination with carboplatin. Data from an ongoing study by the Swedish Lung Cancer Study Group. *Proc ASCO* 2001; **20**: 324a.

97. Kunitoh H, Watanabe K, Ohashi Y et al. Preliminary results of a randomized phase III trial of docetaxel and cisplatin (P) versus vindesine and P in stage IV non small cell lung cancer. *Proc ASCO* 2001; **20**: 323a.

98. Comella P. Phase III trial of cisplatin/gemcitabine with or without vinorelbine or paclitaxel in advanced non-small cell lung cancer. *Semin Oncol* 2001; **28**: 7–10.

99. Danson S, Clemons M, Middleton M et al. A randomised study of gemcitabine with carboplatin versus mitomycin, vinblastine and cisplatin or mitomycin C, ifosfamide and cisplatin as first line chemotherapy in advanced non-small cell lung cancer. *Proc ASCO* 2001; **20**: 322a.

100. Camps C, Alberola V, Provencio M et al. Cisplatin/gemcitabine (CG) vs cisplatin/gemcitabine/vinorelbine (CGV) vs sequential doublets of gemcitabine/vinorelbine followed by ifosfamide/vinorelbine (gv/iv) in advanced non-small cell lung cancer (NSCLC): final results of a Spanish Lung Cancer Group phase III trial (GEPC/98–02). *Eur J Cancer* 2001; **37**: 28.

101. Sculier J, Lafitte J, Paesmans M et al. A three-arms phase III randomised trial comparing combinations of platinum derivatives, ifosfamide and/or gemcitabine in stage IV non-small cell lung cancer

(NSCLC): a European Lung Cancer Working Party study. *Eur J Cancer* 2001; **37**: 29.

102. Rosso R, Cafferata M, Baldini E, De Marinis F. Novel platinum and non-platinum-based triplet regimens in advanced non small cell lung cancer. *Lung Cancer* 2001; **34** (Suppl 1): S41.

103. Souquet P, Tan E, Rodrigues Pereira J et al. A prospective randomized phase III trial comparing vinorelbine and cisplatin versus vinorelbine, ifosfamide and cisplatin in metastatic NSCLC patients: a patient's benefit analysis. *Proc ASCO* 2001; **20**: 335a.

104. Montalar J, Morales S, Maestu I et al. Vinorelbine, ifosfamide and cisplatin as first-line treatment in patients with inoperable non-small cell lung cancer. *Lung Cancer* 2001; **34**: 305–11.

105. Smith IE, O'Brien ME, Talbot DC et al. Duration of chemotherapy in advanced non-small-cell lung cancer: a randomized trial of three versus six courses of mitomycin, vinblastine, and cisplatin. *J Clin Oncol* 2001; **19**: 1336–43.

106. Thompson D, Hainsworth J, Burniss H III, Erland J. Prospective randomized study of four third generation chemotherapy regimens in patients with advanced non-small cell lung cancer: a Minnie Pearl Cancer Research Network trial. *Proc ASCO* 2001; **20**: 314a.

107. Zatloukal P, Petruzelka L, Zemanova M, Kolek V. Gemcitabine plus cisplatin versus gemcitabine plus carboplatin in patients with non-small cell lung cancer stage IIIb and IV: an interim analysis of a randomized trial. *Proc ASCO* 2001; **20**: 337a.

108. Satouchi M, Takada Y, Takeda K et al. Randomized phase II study of docetaxel plus cisplatin versus docetaxel plus irinotecan in advanced non-small cell lung

cancer: a West Japan Thoracic Oncology Group study. *Proc ASCO* 2001; **20**: 329a.

109. Grigorescu A, Draghici I, Gutulescu N, Corlan E. Gemcitabine plus carboplatin (Gcarb) versus cisplatin plus vinblastine (CV) in patients (pts) with stage IIIB and IV non-small cell lung cancer (NSCLC). *Eur J Cancer* 2001; **37**: 21.

110. Chen K, Chen C, Chang W, Lin M. Phase II study of paclitaxel and cisplatin in stage IIIB or IV non-small cell lung cancer. *Proc ASCO* 2001; **20**: 279b.

111. Bando H, Miyata J, Sano T, Sumitomo M. Retrospective analysis of administration of a combination of docetaxel and carboplatin for advanced non-small cell lung cancer. *Anticancer Res* 2001; **21**: 2107–13.

112. Zarogoulidis K, Kontakiotis T, Hatziapostolou P et al. A phase II study of docetaxel and carboplatin in the treatment of non-small cell lung cancer. *Lung Cancer* 2001; **32**: 281–7.

113. Van Kooten M, Coppola F, Jovtis S et al. Feasibility of paclitaxel and carboplatin in advanced non-small cell lung cancer. *Proc ASCO* 2001; **20**: 258b.

114. Novello S, Galli L, Antonuzzo A et al. Phase II study of high-dose paclitaxel and carboplatin in previously untreated, unresectable non-small cell lung cancer. *Lung Cancer* 2001; **34**: 261–9.

115. Glorieux P, Ortmanns P, Marien S et al. Multi-center study of two dose levels of paclitaxel with carboplatin in locally advanced and metastatic non-small cell lung cancer (NSCLC). *Anticancer Res* 2001; **21**: 1487–94.

116. Cremonesi M, Cazzaniga M, Frontini L, Barni S. Carboplatin–vinorelbine: an interesting option for IIIb–IV non-small cell lung cancer treatment. *Proc ASCO* 2001; **20**: 247b.

117. Bretti S, Manzin E, Celano A et al. Low dose carboplatin (AUC 4.5) combined with vinorelbine in the treatment of advanced non-small cell lung cancer: a single institution phase II study. *Oncol Rep* 2001; **8**: 381–5.

118. Terrioux P, Beerblock K, Kanoui A, Colin P. Final results of a GERCOR phase I/II study in chemonaive patients with advanced non small cell lung cancer treated with a bimonthly gemcitabine plus cisplatin regimen. *Proc ASCO* 2001; **20**: 263b.

119. Lee J, Zang D, Byun J et al. Phase II study with paclitaxel and cisplatin chemotherapy as a primary treatment in patients with advanced non-small cell lung cancer. *Proc ASCO* 2001; **20**: 284b.

120. Ho J, Tan E, Wang C et al. Preliminary results of a multi-centre Asian trial of docetaxel and cisplatin in advanced non-small cell lung cancer. *Proc ASCO* 2001; **20**: 238b.

121. Douillard JY, Lerouge D, Monnier A et al. Combined paclitaxel and gemcitabine as first-line treatment in metastatic non-small cell lung cancer: a multicentre phase II study. *Br J Cancer* 2001; **84**: 1179–84.

122. Isla D, Rosell R, Sanchez JJ et al. Phase II trial of paclitaxel plus gemcitabine in patients with locally advanced or metastatic non-small-cell lung cancer. *J Clin Oncol* 2001; **19**: 1071–7.

123. Laack E, Mende T, Benk J et al. Gemcitabine and vinorelbine as first-line chemotherapy for advanced non-small cell lung cancer: a phase II trial. *Eur J Cancer* 2001; **37**: 583–90.

124. Belani CP. Interim analysis of a phase II study of induction weekly paclitaxel/carboplatin regimens followed by maintenance weekly paclitaxel for advanced and metastatic non-small cell lung

cancer. *Semin Oncol* 2001; **28**: 14–16.

125. Belani C, Barstis J, Perry M et al. Phase II multicenter randomized trial of weekly paclitaxel (P) administered in combination with carboplatin followed by maintenance P versus observation for patients with advanced and metastatic non-small cell lung cancer. *Proc ASCO* 2001; **20**: 323a.

126. Jagasia MH, Langer CJ, Johnson DH et al. Weekly irinotecan and cisplatin in advanced non-small cell lung cancer: a multicenter phase II study. *Clin Cancer Res* 2001; **7**: 68–73.

127. Edelman M, Clark J, Chansky K et al. Randomized phase II trial of sequential chemotherapy in advanced non-small cell lung cancer (SWOG 9806): carboplatin/gemcitabine followed by paclitaxel or cisplatin/vinorelbine followed by docetaxel. *Proc ASCO* 2001; **20**: 314a.

128. Depierre A, Quoix E, Mercier M, Breton J. Maintenance chemotherapy in advanced non-small cell lung cancer: a randomized study of vinorelbine versus observation in patients responding to induction therapy. *Proc ASCO* 2001; **20**: 309a.

129. The Elderly Lung Cancer Vinorelbine Italian Study Group. Effects of vinorelbine on quality of life and survival of elderly patients with advanced non-small-cell lung cancer. *J Natl Cancer Inst* 1999; **91**: 66–72.

130. Lanza R, DiGirolamo B, Scirocchi R et al. Vinorelbine as first-line chemotherapy in elderly patients with advanced-metastatic non small cell lung cancer (NSCLC): preliminary result of a phase II study. *Ann Oncol* 2001; **12**(Suppl 4): 69.

131. Galli L, Tibaldi C, Ricci S et al. Chemotherapy with gemcitabine in elderly patients (or in patients not candidate for a cisplatin regimen) with advanced NSCLC: a multi-

center phase II study. *Ann Oncol* 2001; **12**(Suppl 4): 63.

132. Gridelli C, Perrone F, Cigolari S et al. The MILES (Multicenter Italian Lung Cancer in the Elderly Study) phase 3 trial: gemcitabine + vinorelbine vs vinorelbine and vs gemcitabine in elderly advanced NSCLC patients. *Proc ASCO* 2001; **20**: 308a.

133. Kelly K, Giaritta S, Hayes S et al. Should older patients (pts) receive combination chemotherapy for advanced stage non-small cell lung cancer (NSCLC)? An analysis of Southwest Oncology trials 9509 and 9308. *Proc ASCO* 2001; **20**: 329a.

134. Hensing TA, Socinski MA, Schell MJ et al. Age does not alter toxicity or survival for patients (pts) with stage IIIB/IV non-small cell lung cancer (NSCLC) treated with carboplatin (C) and paclitaxel (P). *Proc ASCO* 2001; **20**: 346a.

135. Imperatori L, Lippe P, Laici G et al. Weekly cisplatin (P) and vinorelbine (V) is active and manageable in advanced non-small cell lung cancer (ANSCLC) elderly or poor performance status (PS) patients (PTS). *Ann Oncol* 2001; **12**(Suppl 4): 68.

136. McKay C, Hainsworth J, Burris H et al. Weekly docetaxel/gemcitabine in the treatment of elderly patients (pts) with advanced non-small cell lung cancer (NSCLC): a Minnie Pearl Cancer Research Network phase II trial. *Proc ASCO* 2001; **20**: 260b.

137. Zinner R, Glisson B, Pisters K et al. Cisplatin and gemcitabine combined with herceptin in patients (pt) with her2 overexpressing, untreated, advanced, non-small-cell lung cancer (NSCLC): a phase II trial. *Eur J Cancer* 2001; **37**: 154.

138. Krug L, Miller V, Crapanzano J et al. Randomized phase II trial of trastuzumab plus either weekly docetaxel or paclitaxel in previ-

ously untreated advanced non-small cell lung cancer. *Proc ASCO* 2001; **20**: 333a.

139. Langer C, Adak S, Thor A et al. Phase II Eastern Cooperative Oncology Group pilot study of paclitaxel, carboplatin, and trastuzumab in HER-2/*neu* (+) advanced non-small cell lung cancer: early analysis of E2598. *Lung Cancer* 2001; **34**(Suppl 1): S31.

140. Yuen A, Halsey J, Fisher G, Advani R. Phase I/II trial of ISIS 3521, an antisense inhibitor of PKC-α, with carboplatin and paclitaxel in non-small cell lung cancer. *Proc ASCO* 2001; **20**: 309a.

141. Smylie M, Mercier R, Aboulafia A et al. Phase III study of the matrix metalloprotease inhibitor prinomastat in patients having advanced non-small cell lung cancer. *Proc ASCO* 2001; **20**: 307a.

142. Johnson D, DeVore R, Kabbinavar F et al. Carboplatin + paclitaxel + RhuMab–VEGF may prolong survival in advanced non-squamous lung cancer. *Proc ASCO* 2001; **20**: 315a.

143. Shepherd F, Fossella FV, Lynch T et al. Docetaxel (Taxotere) shows survival and quality-of-life benefits in the second-line treatment of non-small cell lung cancer: a review of two phase III trials. *Semin Oncol* 2001; **28**(1 Suppl 2): 4–9.

144. van Putten J, Baas P, Codrington H et al. Activity of single-agent gemcitabine as second-line treatment after previous chemotherapy or radiotherapy in advanced non-small-cell lung cancer. *Lung Cancer* 2001; **33**: 289–98.

145. Kosmas C, Tsavaris N, Vadiaka M et al. Gemcitabine and docetaxel as second-line chemotherapy for patients with nonsmall cell lung carcinoma who fail prior paclitaxel plus platinum-based regimens. *Cancer* 2001; **92**: 2902–10.

146. Spiridonidis C, Laufman LR, Carman L et al. Second-line chemotherapy for non-small cell lung cancer with monthly docetaxel and weekly gemcitabine: a phase II trial. *Ann Oncol* 2001; **12**: 89–94.

147. Agelaki S, Bania H, Kouroussis C et al. Vinorelbine-based regimens as salvage treatment in patients with advanced non-small cell lung cancer: two parallel multicenter phase II trials. *Oncology* 2001; **60**: 235–41.

8
Mesothelioma

The incidence of mesothelioma continues to increase globally. In the vast majority of cases, it is an incurable tumor that generally occurs following heavy occupational exposure to asbestos. In 2001, Carbone and Testa[1] published a study in which they claimed that there is also a genetic susceptibility to mesothelioma – at least in the Cappadocian region of Turkey – but these conclusions have been disputed strongly by Saracci and Simonato,[2] who have reviewed the literature on the topic.

According to the most recent classification by the World Health Organization/International Association for the Study of Lung Cancer (WHO/IASLC) of lung and pleural tumors, the latter can be classified as epithelioid (50%), sarcomatoid, or desmoplastic biphasic mesothelioma, of which the epithelial tumors have been shown to have a better prognosis than the others. Differentiation between malignant mesothelioma and other forms of cancer, particularly adenocarcinoma, is often difficult, and histochemistry and immunochemistry are important tools in the differentiation, as summarized by the WHO/IASLC Pathology Panel (Table 8.1). Radiography of the chest and computed tomography (CT) remain the key procedures when determining the extent of the disease and evaluation of the diaphragm and mediastinum. Radiologic manifestations tend to be those of pleural effusions and/or pleural thickening. Pleural effusions are initially investigated by thoracocentesis, but the positive diagnosis by pleural fluid cytology is rather low. Pleural biopsy with the presence of pleural effusion has traditionally been performed without image guidance, but in some patients, thoracoscopic biopsy is needed to detect malignant pleural disease, including mesothelioma.

Adams et al[3] reported that a correct histologic diagnosis of malignant mesothelioma can be made by percutaneous image-guided cutting needle biopsy of the pleura with 86% sensitivity and 100% specificity, based on a study of 18 patients. The complications included one chest wall hematoma and a small hemoptysis. For the biopsies, 14- and 18-gauge cutting needles were used, and biopsy guidance was by ultrasound in 6 patients and by CT in 15. Various markers, such as the CYFRA 21–1 tumor marker and carcinoembryonic antigen (CEA), have been assessed as diagnostic tools that could be complementary to cytology in the diagnosis of malignant mesothelioma.[4] CEA and CYFRA 21–1 in the pleural effusions (PEs) and serum in 106 patients (benign

Table 8.1 Immunohistochemistry of pleural lesions[a,b]

Diagnostic problem	Keratins (LMW/HMW)	CEA	B72.3	Leu-M1	BER-EP4	EMA HMFG-2	Vimentin	Actin
I Mesothelial hyperplasia versus	+ to ++	–	–	–	–	–/+	–/+	–
epithelioid mesothelioma versus	+ to ++	–/+	–/+	–/+	–/+	+ (membrane)	+	–/+
metastatic carcinoma (usually adenocarcinoma)	+ to ++	+	+	+	+	+ (cytoplasm)	–/+	–
II Fibrous pleuritis versus	+	–	–	–	–	–/+	+	+
sarcomatoid mesothelioma versus	+	–	–	–	–	–/+	+	+/–
sarcoma (primary or metastatic)	+/–	–	–	–	–	–	+	*

LMW, low molecular weight; HMW, high molecular weight; CEA, carcinoembryonic antigen; EMA, epithelial membrane antigen; HMGF, human milk fat globulin; –, negative; –/+, usually negative; +/–, occasionally positive; +, usually positive; ++, strongly positive; *, depends on subtype.

[a] Adapted from Banks DE, Wang M-I, Parker JE. Asbestos exposure, asbestosis, and lung cancer. *Chest* 1999; 115: 320–2.

[b] Until recently, there has been no immunohistochemical stain that is positive in mesotheliomas and negative in other lesions. HBME-1, calretinin, and thrombomodulin have shown some promise as being mesothelioma-specific antibodies, but none is as yet widely accepted.

lesions, 34; bronchogenic and metastatic carcinoma, 40; mesothelioma, 32) were measured by immunoassays. In all neoplastic PEs, CYFRA 21–1 and CEA sensitivities were 78% and 30.6%, respectively, with specificities of 80% and 91%, respectively. The sensitivities of CYFRA 21–1 and CEA in patients with mesothelioma were 87.5% and 3.1%, respectively. The results of the CYFRA 21–1 assay were positive in 17 of 19 cases of mesothelioma with a negative or uncertain cytology. The association of tumor marker assay and cytology allowed a correct diagnosis in 30 of 32 cases of mesothelioma (93.7%). Accordingly, an elevated CYFRA 21–1 level with a low CEA level is highly suggestive of mesothelioma, whereas high levels of CEA alone or high levels of both the markers suggest a diagnosis of malignant PE, excluding mesothelioma.

With respect to detailed staging, a new system was devised by the Mesothelioma Interest Group (Table 8.2).

In 2001, angiogenesis, as assessed by microvessel density (MVD), was identified, using multivariate Cox analysis, as an independent prognostic factor according to the European Organization for Research and Treatment of Cancer (EORTC) prognostic scoring system ($p = 0.006$),[5] but not to the Cancer and Leukemia Group B (CALGB) scoring system ($p = 0.1$). The conclusions were based on histochemical studies of 104 surgically resected malignant mesothelioma samples using an anti-CD34 monoclonal antibody. Other independent indicators of poor prognosis in multivariate analysis were non-epithelial cell type ($p = 0.002$) and performance status greater than zero ($p = 0.003$).

Other immunohistochemical examinations have been performed, for instance to evaluate catalase expression, both in non-malignant healthy pleura and in tumor tissue of 32 mesothelioma patients.[6] A higher catalase expression in mesothelioma was detected in 75%, versus 0% in non-malignant cells. Higher catalase expression in mesothelioma was associated with a better prognosis.

Other investigators have by immunohistochemistry found that 22 of 30 human mesothelioma tissue samples expressed significantly increased levels of fatty acid synthase (FAS) compared with normal tissues, including mesothelium, and suggest that FAS may be an effective target for pharmacological therapy in a high proportion of human mesotheliomas.[7]

TREATMENT

Treatment of malignant mesothelium remains disappointing regardless of the type of therapy. Radical surgery, such as extrapleural pneumonectomy, should be applied only for the rare patients presenting with localized disease. Surgery has, however, also been attempted as a palliative debulking procedure in malignant mesothelioma, with data being presented by Martin-Ucar et al[8] from the UK. In a prospective study, 51 consecutive patients presenting with malignant mesothelioma underwent palliative surgical debulking for symptomatic relief.

Table 8.2   International TNM staging system for diffuse malignant pleural mesothelioma according to the International Mesothelioma Interest Group[a]

T1	T1a: Tumor limited to the ipsilateral parietal pleura, including mediastinal and diaphragmatic pleura. No involvement of the visceral pleura T1b: Tumor involving the ipsilateral parietal pleura, including mediastinal and diaphragmatic pleura. Scattered foci of tumor also involving the visceral pleura
T2	Tumor involving each of the ipsilateral pleural surfaces (parietal, mediastinal, diaphragmatic, and visceral pleura), with at least one of the following features: • involvement of the diaphragmatic muscle • confluent visceral pleural tumor (including the fissures) or extension of tumor from visceral pleural into the underlying pulmonary parenchyma
T3	Describes locally advanced but potentially resectable tumor. Tumor involving all of the ipsilateral pleural surfaces, with at least one of the following features: • involvement of the endothoracic fascia • extension into the mediastinal fat • solitary, completely resectable focus of tumor extending into the soft tissue of the chest wall • non-transmural involvement of the pericardium
T4	Describes locally advanced, technically unresectable tumor. Tumor involving all of the ipsilateral pleural surfaces, with at least one of the following features: • diffuse extension or multifocal masses of tumor in the chest wall, with or without local rib destruction • direct transdiaphragmatic extension of tumor in the peritoneum • direct extension of tumor to the contralateral pleura • direct extension of tumor in one or more mediastinal organs • direct extension of tumor into the spine • tumor extending through to the internal surface of the pericardium, with or without a pericardial effusion; or tumor involving the myocardium

N: lymph nodes

NX	Regional lymph nodes cannot be assessed
N0	No regional or hilar
N1	Ipsilateral or hilar lymph nodes positive
N2	Mediastinal or ipsilateral internal mammary lymph nodes positive
N3	Contralateral mediastinal, supraclavicular, or contralateral internal mammary lymph nodes positive

M: metastases

MX	Presence of metastases cannot be assessed
M0	No distant metastases
M1	Distant metastases

Stage

Stage IA	T1aN0M0	Stage III	Any T3M0
Stage IB	T1bN0M0		Any N1M0
			Any N2M0
Stage II	T2N0M0	Stage IV	Any T4 or N3 or M1

[a] Reproduced from Travis WD, Colby TV, Corrin B et al (eds). Histological typing of lung and pleural tumours. In: *WHO International Histological Classification of Tumours*, 3rd edn. Berlin: Springer-Verlag, 1999.

The treatment aims were pleural drainage, lung re-expansion, pleurodesis, and pleural debulking for symptom control. If the lung re-expanded after drainage of the effusion, a subtotal parietal pleurectomy was performed via video-assisted thoracic surgery (VATS). If the lung remained entrapped, a parietal and visceral decortication using VATS or thoracotomy was performed. The changes in subjective dyspnea and pain scores were recorded at 6 weeks and at 3, 6, and 12 months after surgery. Morbidity included postoperative empyema in two patients and prolonged air-leak in five patients. Overall significant symptomatic benefit was obtained up to 3 months after surgery, but subsequently increasing mortality offset these benefits. Epithelial cell type and absence of weight loss prior to surgery were found to predict longer survival and successful symptom control.

Research pertaining to drug resistance in malignant mesothelioma was also published in 2001. Soini et al[9] evaluated immunohistochemical expression of P-glycoprotein (P-gp) and multidrug-resistance proteins 1 and 2 (MRP1 and MRP2) in 36 cases of malignant mesothelioma and in samples from normal mesothelium. P-gp immunopositivity was found in 61%, MRP1 immunopositivity in 58%, and MRP2 positivity in 33% of cases. Normal mesothelium did not express these multidrug-resistance proteins. There was a significant association between P-gp and MRP2 ($p = 0.022$) expression. Regardless of their expression, no association with patient survival was seen, suggesting that the primary drug resistance of malignant mesotheliomas is not solely dependent on P-gp or MRP expression or function.

Results using single agents, such as liposomal daunorubicin,[10] gemcitabine, ranpirnase (a novel antitumor ribonuclease), and interleukin-2 (IL-2) immunotherapy are presented in Table 8.3. The response rates in all four phase II trials, which included between 14 and 81 evaluable patients, were disappointing, with response rates for the three first agents being 0%, 0%, and 3%,[10-13] with a median survival of 4.7 months for the gemcitabine patients and 6 months for the ranpirnase patients. The results of immunotherapy using repeated intrapleural instillation of IL-2 were somewhat more encouraging. Toxicity with intrapleural IL-2 consisted of grade 3 fever in 19%. Tumor objective response using WHO criteria, evaluated by CT, occurred in 7 patients (1 complete and 6 patient responses), while 10 achieved steady disease and 14 progressed. The median overall survival was 15 months (range 5–39 months) in all patients. These results warrant further randomized studies with IL-2.

The experience with combination chemotherapy is shown in Table 8.4. Overall, the response rates are higher than with single agents, varying from 16% to 38%, but with overlapping 95% confidence intervals. The median survival rates are also quite similar: 9.3, 9.6, 10.5, and 17.5 months. Two of the trials include two- and three-drug combinations, respectively, using classical

Table 8.3	Single agents for mesothelioma: phase II trials						
Treatment	Dose/ schedule	No. of patients	No. of responders[a]			Response rate (%)[b]	Comments	Ref
			CR	PR	Total			
Liposomal daunorubicin	120 mg/m^2 i.v. q3wks	14	0	0	0	0 (0–23)	–	10
Gemcitabine	1500 mg/m^2 i.v. q3wks	18	0	0	0	0 (0–18)	Median survival 4.7 months; 1-year survival rate 24%	11
Ranpirnase	480 µg/m^2 weekly	81	0	4	3	4 (1–12)	Median survival 6 months for intent-to-treat group and 8.3 months for treatment target group	12
IL-2 immunotherapy	9 × 10^6 IU intrapleurally twice weekly for 4 weeks	31	1	6	7	22 (9–41)	Median survival 15 months (range 3–39 months)	13

[a] CR, complete response; PR, partial response.
[b] 95% confidence intervals in parentheses.

cytostatic agents, while interferon-α2b (IFN-α2b) and *Mycobacterium vaccae* (SRL172) were added to combination chemotherapy in the studies by the Italian Lung Cancer Task Force and by Mendes et al[17] from the UK. The latter trial combined chemotherapy with intratumor/intrapleural SRL172, achieving a response rate of 33%. The proposed rationale behind this combination was that the chemotherapy, although slightly immunosuppressive, could cause the in vivo release and subsequent presentation of tumor antigens and trigger a tumor-specific response by the immune system when boosted by an immunomodulator such as SRL172.

Table 8.4   Combination chemotherapy for mesothelioma

Treatment[a]	No. of patients	No. of responders			Response rate (%)[b]	Comments	Ref
		CR	PR	Total			
Gemcitabine + cisplatin	25	0	4	4	16 (1–31)	Median survival 9.6 months	14
Mitoxantrone + methotrexate + mitomycin C	22	1	6	7	32 (12–51)	Median survival 13.5 months	15
Cisplatin + doxorubicin + IFN-α2b	35	0	0	10	29 (15–47)	Median survival 9.3 months 1 year: 45% 2 year: 34%	16
Mitomycin C + cisplatin + vinblastine + (SRL172)	15	0	0	6	37.5 (16–67)	Median survival 10.5 months	17
Ifosfamide + carboplatin + etoposide + hyperthermia[c]	15	0	5	5	33 (11–62)	Abstract	18

[a] IFN, interferon; SRL172, *Mycobacterium vaccae*.
[b] 95% confidence intervals in parentheses.
[c] 41.8°C (× 60 minutes) radiant-heat whole-body hyperthermia (WBH).

REFERENCES

1. Carbone M, Testa JR. Genetic susceptibility and familial malignant mesothelioma. *Lancet* 2001; **357**: 1804.

2. Saracci R, Simonato L. Familial malignant mesothelioma. *Lancet* 2001; **358**: 1813.

3. Adams RF, Gray W, Davies RJO, Gleeson FV. Percutaneous image-guided cutting needle biopsy of the pleura in the diagnosis of malignant mesothelioma. *Chest* 2001; **120**: 1798–1802.

4. Paganuzzi M, Onetto M, Marroni P et al. Diagnostic value of CYFRA 21–1 tumor marker and CEA in pleural effusion due to mesothelioma. *Chest* 2001; **119**: 1138–42.

5. Edwards JG, Cox G, Andi A et al. Angiogenesis is an independent prognostic factor in malignant mesothelioma. *Br J Cancer* 2001; **85**: 863–8.

6. Kahlos K, Soini Y, Sormunen R et al. Expression and prognostic significance of catalase in malignant mesothelioma. *Cancer* 2001; **91**: 1349–57.

7. Gabrielson EW, Pinn ML, Testa JR, Kuhajda FP. Increased fatty acid

synthase is a therapeutic target in mesothelioma. *Clin Cancer Res* 2001; 7: 153–7.

8. Martin-Ucar AE, Edwards JG, Rengajaran A et al. Palliative surgical debulking in malignant mesothelioma. Predictors of survival and symptom control. *Eur J Cardio-Thorac Surg* 2001; 20: 1117–21.

9. Soini Y, Järvinen K, Kaarteenaho-Wiik R, Kinnula V. The expression of P-glycoprotein and multidrug resistance proteins 1 and 2 (MRP1 and MRP2) in human malignant mesothelioma. *Ann Oncol* 2001; 12: 1239–45.

10. Steele JPC, O'Doherty CA, Shamash J et al. Phase II trial of liposomal daunorubicin in malignant pleural mesothelioma. *Ann Oncol* 2001; 12: 497–99.

11. Kindler HL, Millard F, Herndon JE II et al. Gemcitabine for malignant mesothelioma: a phase II trial by the Cancer and Leukemia Group B.

12. Mikulski SM, Costanzi JJ, Vogelzang NJ et al. Phase II trial of a single weekly intravenous dose of ranpirnase in patients with unresectable malignant mesothelioma. *J Clin Oncol* 2001; 20: 274–81.

13. Castagneto B, Zai S, Mutti L et al. Palliative and therapeutic activity of IL-2 immunotherapy in unresectable malignant pleural mesothelioma with pleural effusion. Results of a phase II study on 31 consecutive patients. *Lung Cancer* 2001; 31: 303–10.

14. van Haarst JMW, Baas P, Manegold C et al. Multicentre phase II study of gemcitabine and cisplatin in malignant pleural mesothelioma. *Br J Cancer* 2002; 96: 342–5.

15. Pinto C, Marino A, Guaraldi M et al. Combination chemotherapy with mitoxantrone, methotrexate, and mitomycin (MMM regimen) in malignant pleural mesothelioma. *Am J Clin Oncol* 2001; 24: 143–7.

16. Parra HS, Tixi L, Latteri F et al. Combined regimen of cisplatin, doxorubicin, and α-2b interferon in the treatment of advanced malignant pleural mesothelioma. *Cancer* 2001; 92: 650–6.

17. Mendes R, O'Brien MER, Mitra A et al. Clinical and immunological assessment of *Mycobacterium vaccae* (SRL172) with chemotherapy in patients with malignant mesothelioma. *Br J Cancer* 2002; 96: 336–41.

18. Bakhshandeh A, Bruns I, Eberhardt K et al. A Systemic Hyperthermia Oncology Working Group trial: ifosfamide (IFO), carboplatin (CBDCA) and etoposide (VP-16) combined with aquatherm induced 41.8°C whole body hyperthermia (WBH) for adult patients with malignant pleural mesothelioma. *Proc ASCO* 2001; 20: 341a (Abst 1361).

9
Summary

A short summary of the management of small cell lung cancer (SCLC), non-small cell lung cancer (NSCLC), and mesothelioma is given in this chapter, based on the evidence from randomized trials, even though it should be realized that patients included in clinical trials are not representative of the patient population as a whole. Additional information on the management of lung cancer can be found in review articles published during the last year.[1-6]

SMALL CELL LUNG CANCER

Limited disease

For the rare patient who presents with stage I disease, surgical resection followed by postoperative chemotherapy is the treatment of choice. The results for SCLC are equivalent to the treatment of stages I and II NSCLC. For the more typical SCLC patient who presents with bulky limited disease, combination chemotherapy, in conjunction with radiotherapy, is the mainstay of treatment. For chemotherapy, etoposide plus cisplatin (EP) has become the most commonly used regimen because of fewer toxic side-effects and at least a similar activity to regimens containing doxorubicin or cyclophosphamide. The combination of carboplatin and etoposide produces similar results as EP and has a more favourable toxicity profile. The optimal dosage of cisplatin has not yet been clearly defined.

Based on meta-analyses, chest irradiation has shown superior results in patients receiving combination chemotherapy and radiotherapy compared with those receiving chemotherapy alone. The optimal timing and dosing of chest irradiation are still uncertain, but there is a tendency to initiate radiotherapy early during the first two courses at total doses of at least 50 Gy. Hyperfractionated radiotherapy given twice a day has yielded superior survival data compared with conventional radiotherapy when combined with EP.

Prophylactic cranial irradiation (PCI) has also been demonstrated to have a statistically significant impact on survival in patients with limited disease who achieve a complete remission, while no such data exist for patients with

135

extensive disease achieving a complete remission. The optimal dose and timing of radiotherapy are again uncertain; most frequently, the total dose does not exceed 30 Gy given in fractions of 2.5 Gy daily.

Extensive disease

A combination of etoposide and cisplatin is again the preferred standard treatment. The replacement of etoposide with irinotecan given together with cisplatin has resulted in significantly better median survivals and 1-year survival rates. Again, carboplatin can be substituted for cisplatin because of its similar activity and fewer mucosal side-effects, even though the myelosuppression is higher. Recent results have indicated that a four-drug combination of etoposide, cisplatin, epirubicin, and cyclophosphamide may be superior to etoposide and cisplatin alone.

With regard to maintenance therapy, the hypothesis has been tested of adding either oral etoposide or topotecan to the treatment regimen in patients demonstrating a response to initial therapy. The results showed a slight improvement with etoposide of median progression-free survival, whereas topotecan did not show any significant difference. The impact of dose intensification remains uncertain; no superior effect has been obtained with intensification of the treatment using shorter intervals between treatments.

None of the phase III trials incorporating new agents has shown superior results compared with classical combinations, such as cisplatin/carboplatin plus etoposide.

In patients presenting with poor prognostic factors, such as performance status 3–4, involvement of the liver and bone marrow, and severe comorbid diseases, the initial dose of chemotherapy should be reduced, and careful monitoring is recommended over the first weeks.

Elderly patients with poor performance status and widespread disease have a substantially higher risk of incurring treatment-related complications, and generally have a poor outcome. Supportive measures alone are often the best option for some of these patients.

Recurrent disease

The treatment options depend on the anatomic site of relapse, symptomatology, and previous treatment. Local relapse in patients without prior chest irradiation is best treated with palliative radiotherapy. Late relapse in patients who initially responded to a platinum-containing regimen should receive the same regimen again. Otherwise, single-agent chemotherapy with, for example, topotecan or combination chemotherapy with cyclophosphamide, doxorubicin, and vincristine is the treatment of choice. Newer agents are being tested in this group of patients either as single agents or in combinations, but are yielding response rates of less than 20%.

NON-SMALL CELL LUNG CANCER

A short summary of the management of NSCLC is given in this section, based on data reported in 2001. Chapter 7 provides detailed information on the current treatment options for patients with this disease.

STAGES I, II, AND RESECTABLE IIIA

Stage I

The standard therapy for stage I NSCLC continues to be complete surgical resection when possible. This should include lobectomy plus sampling of all mediastinal nodal stations or complete lymph node dissection. However, the surgical technique to perform a lobectomy and mediastinal exploration may be changing as experience with minimally invasive surgery grows. Data reviewed in 2001 revealed encouraging results with video-assisted thoracic surgery (VATS) lobectomy and mediastinal sampling or dissection. With minimal invasive surgery becoming popular, the efficacy of minimal resections such as segmentectomy and wedge resection is also being readdressed as smaller tumors (< 1–2 cm) are being identified with spiral computed tomography (CT) scans. Another critical question is the relationship of tumor size to nodal metastasis. Data have been presented suggesting that histology and size may be beneficial in determining nodal risk.

For patients who are medically inoperable, advances in radiotherapy such as three-dimensional (3D) conformal and stereotactic radiosurgery are producing more durable results with decreased toxicity.

Stage IB–IIIA

Adjuvant therapy to surgery, such as radiotherapy or chemotherapy, was assessed in small phase II trials in 2001 with encouraging results. However, there remains pessimism about the possible benefit of adjuvant therapies because the majority of past randomized trials have not shown a survival benefit with this approach. The definitive answer awaits the data from seven recently completed or ongoing randomized phase III trials. Meanwhile, newer strategies with targeted therapies have been implemented.

Alternatively, neoadjuvant therapies are being increasingly used. While large randomized trials investigating this important topic continue to enroll patients, we have learned over the past year that neoadjuvant chemotherapy does not significantly increase surgical morbidity or mortality. Hopefully, this data demonstrating the feasibility of administering neoadjuvant chemotherapy will foster accrual to these large trials.

For patients with operable stage III (N2) disease, the number of lymph nodes involved and the ability to eradicate tumor from the lymph nodes with neoadjuvant therapy were found to be important prognostic factors. Meanwhile, the pivotal question about the role of surgery in the treatment of stage IIIA (N2) disease will be elucidated in 2003 when the results of the Intergroup trial in North America of neoadjuvant chemoradiotherapy followed by surgery versus chemoradiotherapy alone become available. Furthermore as multimodality therapy leads to improved survival for patients with operable NSCLC, an increased frequency of isolated brain metastases have been observed, which must be addressed.

INOPERABLE STAGE III

Current chemoradiotherapy is the standard of care for patients with inoperable stage III NSCLC. However numerous questions remain regarding the optimal means to combine these two modalities and whether there is a benefit of additional therapy before or after chemoradiotherapy. No phase III results were available in 2001 addressing these issues. Randomized phase II trials with newer cytotoxic agents given with concurrent radiation or trials incorporating an induction or consolidation chemotherapy approach failed to show median survivals beyond the standard 17 months in most instances. Trials evaluating altered radiotherapy fractions have also not improved survival. Exciting areas of future research include the roles of 3D conformal radiotherapy, intense modified radiotherapy (IMRT), and the addition of targeted agents, with several agents demonstrating radiosensitization.

STAGE IV (AND IIIB WITH PLEURAL EFFUSION)

Doublet chemotherapy for stage IIIB with pleural effusion and stage IV NSCLC patients with adequate performance status has been shown in multiple randomized studies to improve survival and quality of life, and remains the standard of care. We have spent the last decade determining whether any new platinum-based regimen was superior. Numerous randomized trials clearly found all regimens to be equally efficacious, but to differ in toxicity and cost. Trials presented in 2001 continue to support this finding. Furthermore, data from randomized trials that included a non-platinum regimen were equivalent in efficacy to platinum regimens. No change in the current recommendations for patients with advanced NSCLC occurred in 2001, with a platinum-based doublet remaining as the treatment regimen of choice. While numerous phase II cytotoxic regimens were evaluated, none produced amazing results. Thus, enthusiasm for exploring traditional cytotoxic regimens has dampened, and the focus has switched to targeted therapies.

A variety of targeted agents were evaluated in 2001, including trastuzumab, ISIS-3521, prinomastat, and the anti-VEGF monoclonal antibody RhuMab-

VEGF. Although the results with prinomastat were negative, the encouraging results with all of the other targeted agents have led to the initiation of phase III trials. Another interesting class of agents are the inhibitors of the epidermal growth factor receptor (Iressa, Tarceva, and Erbitux), which have produced responses in heavily pretreated patients and are in phase III trials.

A host of targeted agents are in earlier stages of clinical evaluation, such as Cox-2 inhibitors, the preapoptotic inhibitor exisulind, proteasome inhibitors, targretin, and vaccines. However, we must be cautiously optimistic about targeted therapy, because it brings with it a new set of problems to tackle. Determining clinical and biologic efficacy is a major barrier, and long-term toxicity is ill-defined for most of these agents.

Improving upon the efficacy of second-line docetaxel, investigators have focused on the addition of a second cytotoxic agent. Several small studies showed a favorable survival improvement for doublet therapy, but further investigation is needed. The second-line setting is ideal for evaluating targeted therapies. These agents will undoubtedly be investigated alone or in combination with docetaxel. Doublets have also been explored in the elderly population, but have not demonstrated value over a single agent.

MESOTHELIOMA

Surgery should be considered when mesothelioma remains localized – usually as extrapleural pneumonectomy. Chemotherapy and/or radiotherapy have not yet proved to be effective in preventing local recurrence, nor has the use of photodynamic therapy or intracavitary chemotherapy.

With respect to chemotherapy, quantitative and qualitative overviews of the literature have suggested that cisplatin may have an important role to play in combination therapy. It is also emerging that response rates of 30–40% can be obtained when combining cisplatin with other agents, for example altitrexed and pemitrexed disodium (LY-231514, Alimta). Photodynamic therapy, hyperthermia, and immunotherapy with *Mycobacterium vaccae* combined with chemotherapy have also been tested in phase II trials, but the relatively small numbers of patients in the various trials preclude firm conclusions.

REFERENCES

1. Hoffman PC, Mauer AM, Vokes EE. Lung cancer. *Lancet* 2000; **355**: 479–85.

2. Schiller JC. Current standards of care in small-cell and non-small-cell lung cancer. *Oncology* 2001; **61**(Suppl 1): 3–13.

3. Pastorino U. Lung cancer: diagnosis and surgery. *Eur J Cancer* 2001: 7 (Suppl 7): S75–90.

4. Van Houtte P. The role of radiotherapy and the value of combined treatment in lung cancer. *Eur J Cancer* 2001; 37(Suppl 7): S91–8.

5. Giaccone G. State of the art in systemic treatment of lung cancer. *Eur J Cancer* 2001; **37**(Suppl 7): S99–114.

6. Bunn PA Jr. Novel targeted agents for the treatment of lung cancer. In: *ASCO Educational Book*, 2002; 683–92.

Index

N.B. Combination drugs are shown with components in alphabetical order.